A MEASURE OF JOY

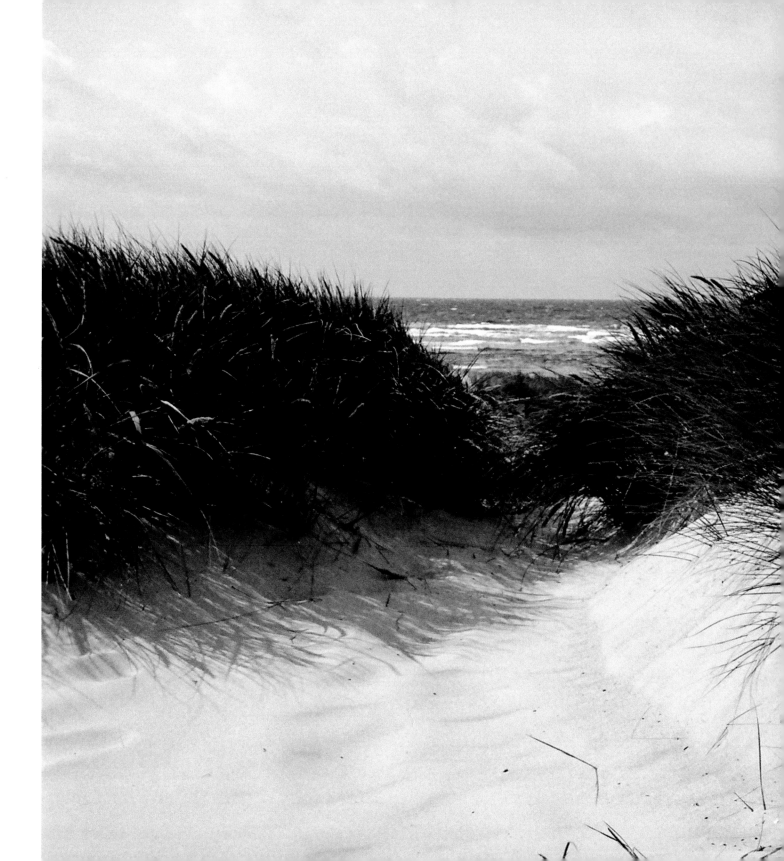

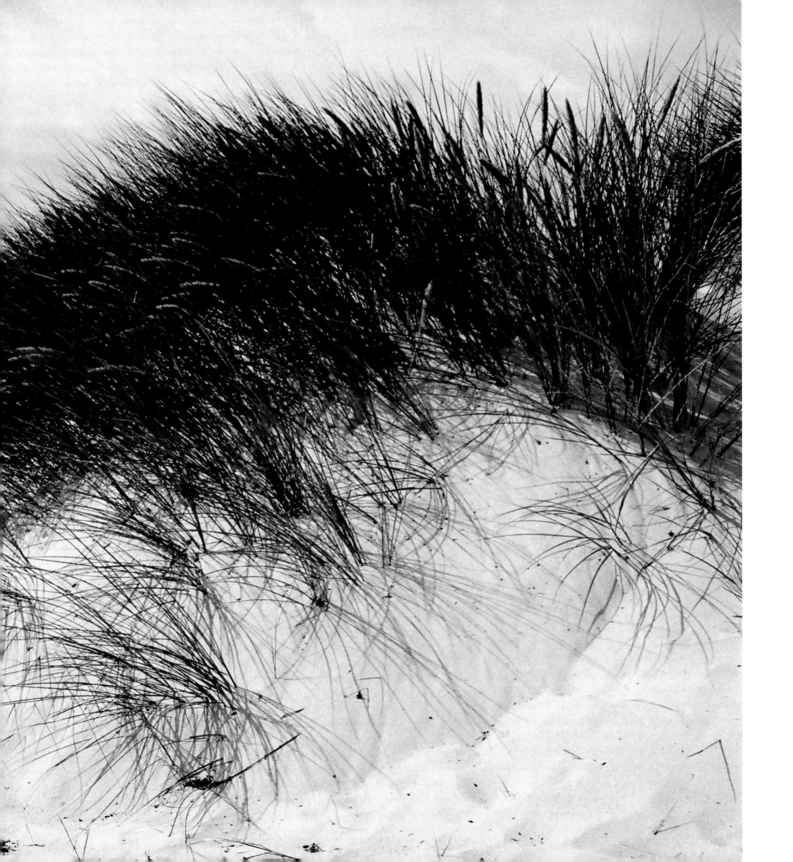

Library of Congress Control Number:
2009927985

ISBN 978-1-934491-13-3

First Edition

Publisher
Fresco Fine Art Publications, llc
Albuquerque, New Mexico
www.frescobooks.com

Copyright ©2009

Design and Production
Fresco Fine Art Publications, llc

Printed in Italy

A MEASURE OF JOY

OPENING TO THE ENERGY OF REIKI

GAY STINNETT

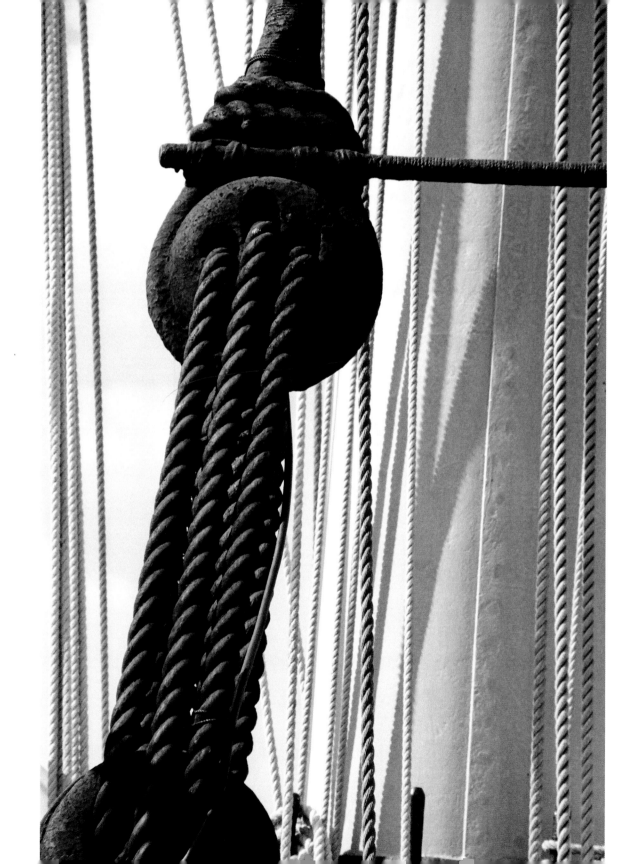

CONTENTS

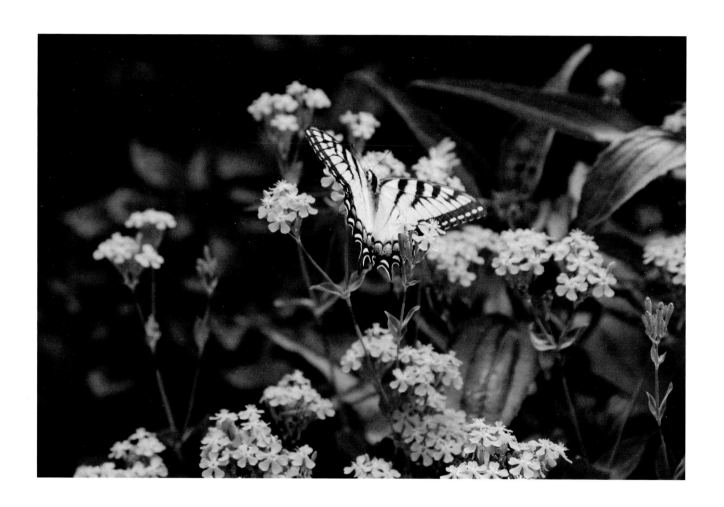

FOR MARY ELEANOR McCREADY KIRK
my mother and my mentor
who opened so many doors

FOREWORD

We are all connected.

Whether through blood, experience, memories, activities, dreams, or thoughts, we are connected to people, animals, nature, and even inanimate objects. Everything we can see, and many things we cannot see, are made of energy. Every thought, emotion, spoken word, every table, tree, or rock—everything is energy.

Energy vibrates at different frequencies and thereby appears—or does not appear—in different ways, whether as music or art, or as dirt or bones. Some vibration resonates, some teaches; some vibration irritates, and some brings joy.

It took many years for me to acknowledge this connection. Rather than begrudging the time it took, I am joyful that I have reached this point. I understand that Reiki is energy and that energy connects everything. Energy changes; energy is constant. Over the years, I have seen Reiki calm, soothe, and bring peace, just as I have seen Reiki energize, focus, and bring joy.

Teaching others to share Reiki is my passion. On this path, I have noticed human traits getting in the way of some students' joy of offering this relaxation therapy. Ego, fear, lack of imagination, timing, or location—so many perceived roadblocks—can appear to practitioners. I wish to de-clutter the connection.

In writing this book, it has been my wish to share stories, with privacy honored, and to offer ideas and hints with Reiki students as well as Reiki recipients. This is my way to offer relaxation and joy, and to share the wondrous gift of Reiki.

After all, we are all connected.

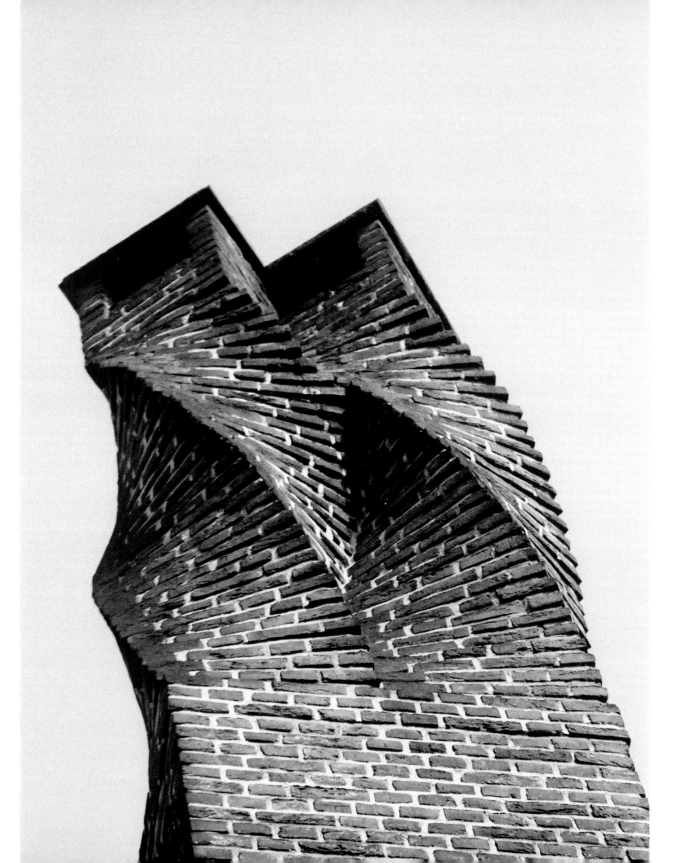

I came from a family with limited heritage and few traditions. Although my parents had four children, my extended family was small, with only one true uncle, a great uncle and the limited offspring of each. A grandmother and step-grandparents rounded out the simple family tree.

There was one tradition that initially threw me a curve ball at the beginning of my life. My mother's side of our family had passed the name "Eleanor" down at least three generations. It's a nice name, one that can mutate depending on personality and age. Ellie, Leana, Norie. A cornucopia of choices awaited the proud bearer of the family's connection.

One might assume that the first daughter would have the family name bestowed upon her, but my parents broke that unwritten rule when I was born. I was named Gay, and the next daughter received the historic Eleanor. Whenever I asked why they skipped over me to award the special family name, I was always assured that they had given great thought to their choice of Gay. In my early questioning, I discovered more logic behind my parents' name choice for a boy, Stephen Paul—"Stephen" after my mother's obstetrician and "Paul" after her brother. So there I was, with a name my parents loved, but one that would cause future struggles.

One can only imagine the challenges that my name has brought to me during my life. Most hearing impaired individuals slip into Kay or Faye, a more neutral interpretation. Many swear they hear Gayle (or Gail). I would hear my name with every "Hey" called out in public conversation, while other possibilities, including "Okay" in a sentence, had my ears perking up and my head swiveling.

Initially, I began with Gay Ann (employing my middle name). A bit Southern, and also confusing, since I became "Gann" to some, as we fast-talking Northerners condensed the moniker that identified that pudgy, freckle-faced redhead.

My grandmother, a former dean of women at a prestigious university, had encountered a "rebel" student by the name of Gay. As a result, for most of my life, she called me Ann, or Ann, Dear (the double name thing again). It was only in her later years that she allowed Gay Ann to appear in written form. By that time, however, I had made yet another name shift.

As I began my teen years, I broke out of the mold (one of many over the years) and took Ann out of the equation. Gay became the cute, sassy name of choice. By that time, I had developed a personality which was full of fun and which took pleasure in the moment. This was also the time during which "gay" took on a new meaning in our society. I spent many a year straightening out my sexual orientation with professors, employers, and men of interest, as blushing became second nature…. "Are you gay (Gay)?" required my response of "Yes, my name is Gay." Today, when introducing myself, I usually shine a smile and say

"Hi, my name is Gay," only occasionally slipping to say (with that same smile) "Hi, I'm Gay."

As each life changing event occurred, I toyed with a name change. My parents said I could change my name at eighteen years of age. Christine was my favorite. But at eighteen, I seemed to have a lot more to do than initiating a name change. I took my husbands' last name(s) at my wedding ceremony(ies) in order to spruce up the Gay thing. At my first wedding rehearsal dinner, my future father-in-law welcomed "Kay" into the family. An easy slip, but it also could have been a reference to the previous girlfriend by that very name. Another blushing event, and one that held more than a misspoken name.

I even attempted Annie during an Internet dating phase. I checked with numerologists and psychics. Some seemed to think my name had nothing to do with my essence, while others claimed that short and sweet Gay was the only way to go.

I had entered the working world with eager anticipation. Some jobs provided anonymity, and names were rarely used. Some careers, such as antique shop owner, allowed for a quirky name in a quirky field. I roamed the world of business without much reaction to my name. After becoming involved in the corporate banking industry, I stiffened my name and signature to "Gay A.," thereby displaying strength, power and stability, or so I believed. At one point, I worked with a fellow lender with the name of Joy. Now that was a happy department!

Over the years in a predominately male work environment, I noticed that many referred to me by my last name, you know, one of the boys. Even a client who had spoken to me by phone, sent written correspondence to "Gary." That rubbed a bit, but, hey, I was one of the boys! And, socially I began to be at peace with my name.

After sailing through many careers, my life path has finally settled. I know now that a desk, office, or business does not dictate my name. Now that I have found my life path, I have also accepted my perfect name.

Most of my employment has contained the core elements of helping others and teaching. Through these experiences, I gained the skills that support my ultimate *raison d'etre*: the sharing of life force energy. I now represent a foundation which promotes Integrative Therapies for the community. My personal path is what is meaningful and is what will hopefully be remembered.

My name has been a conversation starter. My name has brought smiles to most of my clients and patients. My name has helped form my personality. I smile more than many, laugh with abandon, and identify the joy of life with ease. And now, as I begin the path of author, I have no need to agonize over the name under the title. My name is Gay.

The secret of fortune is joy in our hands.
—Ralph Waldo Emerson

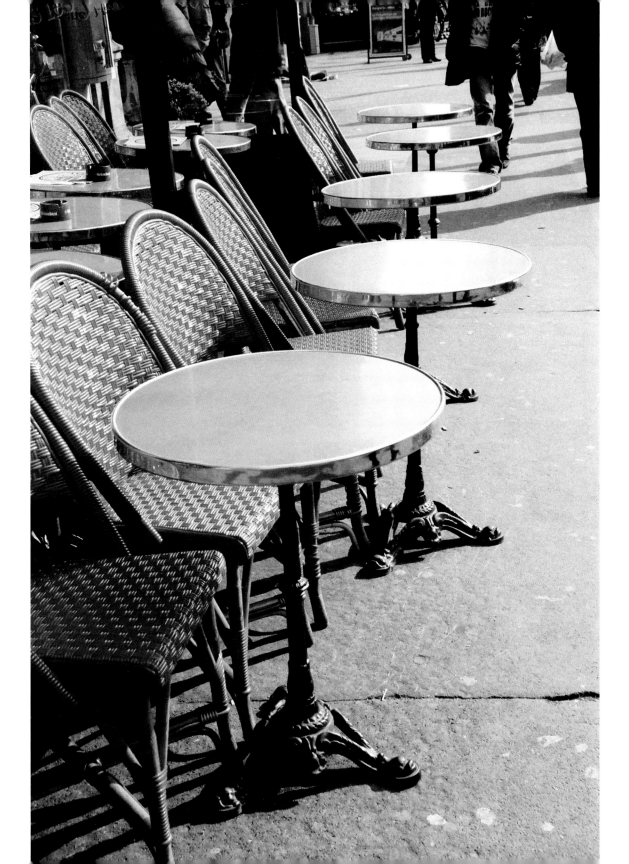

Red hair and freckles allow for individuality more so than blond tresses and porcelain skin. At least that has been my justification for a life that includes marching to a different drummer and dancing to an unheard melody. Mine has been a life that bends rules, avoids structure, and stretches the boundaries.

I created a life of contrasts early, as my parents allowed me to push and explore my world. The fact that I never crawled did not stop me from getting what I wanted. Scooting and reaching began my life, without always using the acceptable methods. I went through my youth walking the fine line of propriety, but always testing it. Although I was aware of the rules and structure, I often enjoyed moments with little conscious regard for consequences.

As an adult, I fell into my careers without much effort. Whatever presented itself that involved joy was my choice. Retail sales allowed me to earn money for fun and frills and to start a savings path that included college. Medical receptionist opportunities opened the exciting world of doctors and cures. Whether as a real estate developer's assistant, small business owner, or banker, I was always involved in the local community as well as in the world at large.

Ever a woman who lived in the moment, as I matured, I noticed a common thread throughout my career. I enjoyed providing service to others. I had an underlying need to help. From offering goodies at the candy counter of a department store to providing financing for a new business, I was (and am) a pleaser. Bringing a smile, a contented sigh, a pleased response—each seemed to soothe my soul.

The hard part was remaining within the confines of a particular job description or regulation attached to a field. The health codes governing the selling of candy were just the beginning of the many structures I was to discover wherever I turned: scheduling busy doctors with just the right amount of time for diagnosis; collecting and remitting sales tax; becoming aware of construction and development codes. The rules always seemed to choke my free spirit.

What appeared to be a frustration with individual employers actually was revealed to be my personal need to "do it a different way." That is acceptable when self-employed or when providing a product that requires no personal contact or regulation attached to its production. It becomes more challenging when attempting to fit into prescribed opportunities. Since I have prided myself with my desire to give back and be of service, I continue to poke, prod, and challenge.

Today I am walking down my perfect path—a path that is not currently universally accepted as the beaten path of life—as a Reiki Master/Teacher.

Reiki pleases, relaxes, and elicits smiles. Reiki heals. Reiki allows your body to be the best it can be. Reiki is completely safe for all ages. It is an energetic modality that promotes relaxation and adjusts naturally to the recipient's needs. Reiki has no side effects. It supports the body's natural ability to heal itself by releasing blocked energy, and thereby relieving pain, facilitating growth, and reducing stress and anxiety.

So, what exactly is this fairly recent technique based on an ancient healing art? Since the late 1800s, scientists, medical professionals, and laypersons have been exploring the sharing of and connection with Universal Life Force Energy. Reiki identifies this energy as perfect and more powerful than anything we may see or know. Traditionally, a practitioner is trained to acknowledge and share this energetic vibration, which itself is a component of everything of which we are aware. Everything is made of energy. All energy vibrates. When we are at our best, whether plant, animal, or inanimate object, we are vibrating as perfectly as we can.

As life demonstrates, we are rarely at our best. We skin a knee, rip a leaf, or crack a surface. At that point, vibrations are blocked, cells are damaged, or molecules are skewed. By becoming "a straw" for Universal Life Force Energy, a practitioner can infuse the intended recipient (including himself) with this perfect energy that allows the recipient to be at his or its best.

More rules, traditions, and limitations? Just the opposite! The beauty of Reiki is that, although there are prescribed positions, timing, and teachings, these suggestions may be adjusted to fit time, place, and condition. A limited time schedule, a public space, and even one hand can share this calming energy. In a crowd or on a massage table, with soft music or a plane's accelerating engines, a simple touch or even sent from a distance, Reiki can be shared. Intention and caring are the components needed and those can be shared anywhere, at any time.

At last I have found a place for my individuality, one that accepts and embraces my differences, and supports the integrity of my path of service.

Never let anyone steal your joy.
—Mike Richards

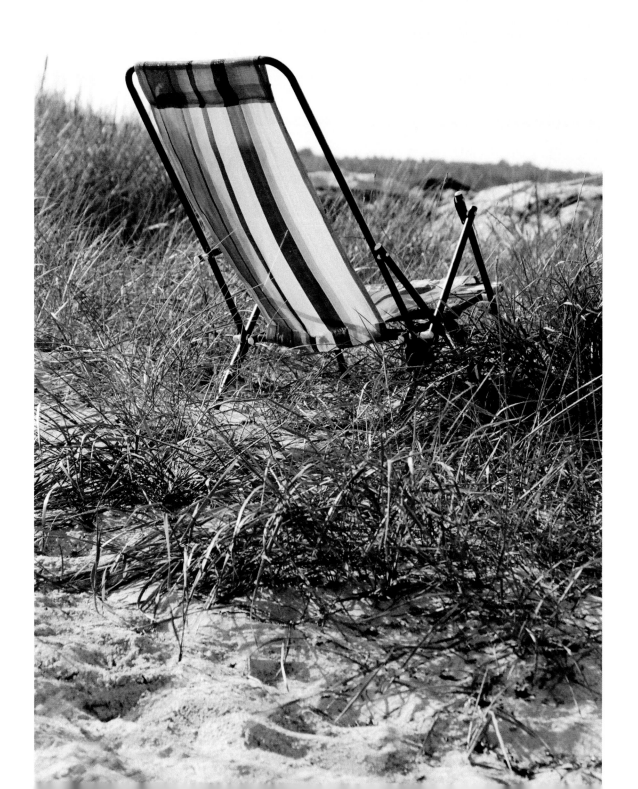

THE AWAKENING

I am a Virgo. In the past my Virgo traits were many and obvious: structured, stubborn, organized, impatient, detailed. I most recently excelled in the banking industry, one that was tailor-made for a Virgo. Perhaps that explains my success.

I have my sisters to thank for my introduction into the world of Integrative Therapies. While I was saving the world, one loan at a time, my two sisters were saving us, one energy client at a time. As I stuck to my structured, rigid regulations, they floated in the magical world of healing. When around them, if I could have worn a cloak to protect me from that world, I would have. Luckily we respected one another's beliefs and co-existed peacefully, even allowing for a raised eyebrow or two.

As my mother ended her days, my sisters supported the idea of offering massage and Reiki to her with a local practitioner. A few times a month my mother would drift away from her pain and fear into a calm and peaceful cocoon. I appreciated the results, but did not give the cause much thought.

When my sisters visited my mother, Reiki, intention, and prayers were offered. I was a more action-driven individual. I made lists and checked off the completion of tasks. We each handled the situation in the best way we could.

My mother entered hospice and a burden was lifted from my shoulders. Calm, competent professionals joined with me in caring for her. I cannot speak highly enough about the hospice concept, and because of that rewarding experience, I am an avid volunteer today.

The day before my mother passed, my whole family was together with her and bid farewell as a group. It was emotional and touching. The following day, predetermined meetings and responsibilities took some away. My East Coast sister and I remained in vigil. We left the hired caregiver in charge late that afternoon as we slipped away to have our nails done. Within a half hour, the caregiver called crying, to tell us that our mother was gone. It was almost as if she waited to leave on her journey alone, without familiar support.

We rushed back to take up our posts and dutifully called hospice. The nurse on call was new to our family, but had certainly been sent by a higher power as the perfect companion to sort out the next steps. As she assessed our situation, she mentioned that she was a Reiki practitioner as was my sister and they began bonding. I wandered away, moving around the room, getting used to the silence of the quieted oxygen machine and to hearing my own breathing. I paid little attention to the murmurings of plans and responsibilities.

My sister was impressed by her discovery of the interest in Reiki during hospice and, in honor of my mother, donated funds to continue hospice's work and in addition, set up a Reiki program. At the same time, she offered to teach me this calm, soothing relaxation technique. Although I was hesitant, I wanted to support her first class and I agreed to attend.

I became a born-again Reiki practitioner. I dragged any friend (and at times mere acquaintances) to my home to share this powerful gift. I was instrumental in developing the local hospice Reiki program, eventually providing Reiki to any employee or volunteer interested in discovering the potential of this tool. Later, I was one of the teachers used by hospice to train staff and volunteers. I continue to provide Reiki to patients.

I will also tell you that our mother's final hospice nurse has become a close friend, mentor, and supporter. She embodies all that is joyful in Reiki, hospice, and life.

Over the years, I have watched my more strident Virgo traits fade as my energy has changed. I am perfecting the "live in the moment" mantra I have adhered to for most of my life. I have let go of those important lists, demands, and "shoulds." I have simplified and become more aware. Today I am quieter, slower, and smell more roses. I do not give total credit to age.

I am awakening.

Joy is but the sign
that creative emotion is fulfilling its purpose.
—Charles Du Bos

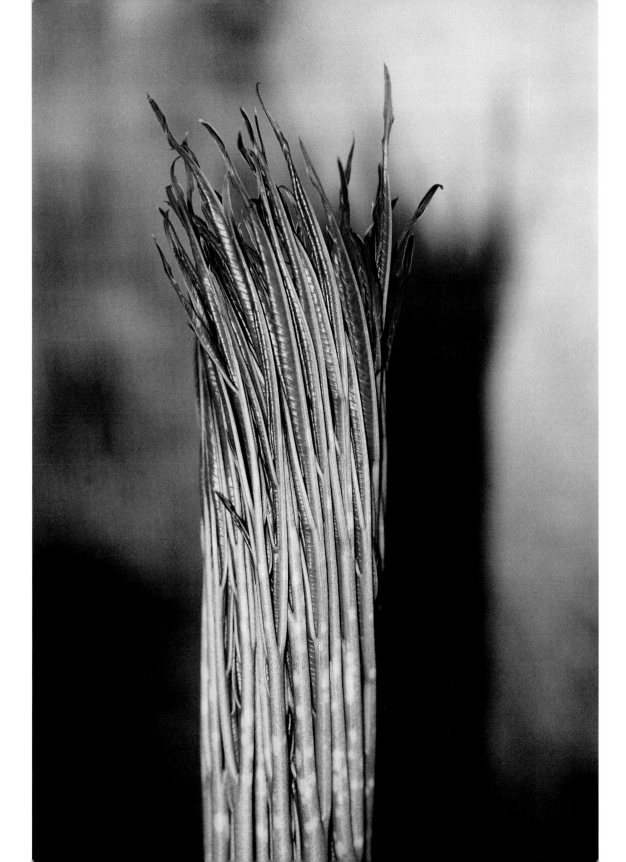

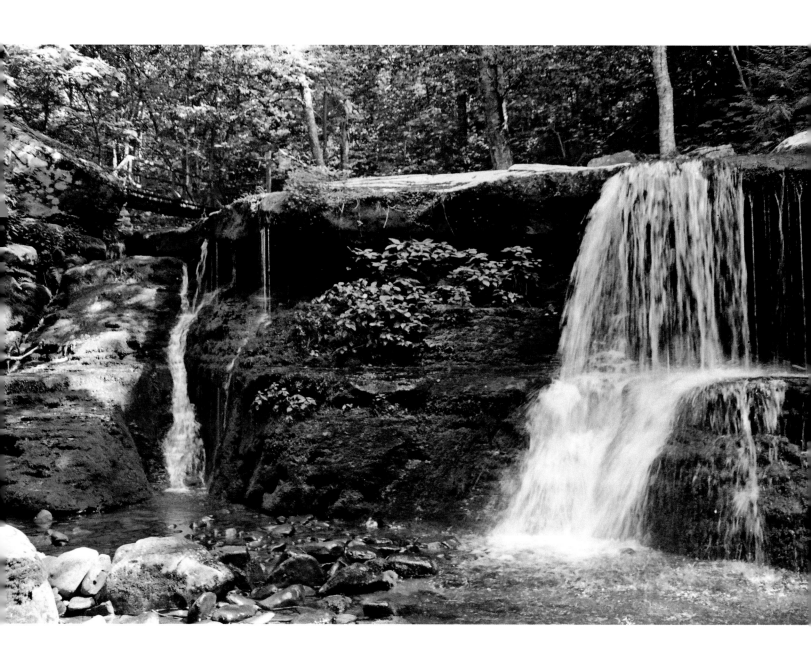

At one point during the unfolding of my path, I was asked to explain Reiki and its use with patients, to a group of nurses. Any group of medical professionals can appear daunting when attempting to share a newly resurfaced tool for enhanced patient care. Medical professionals have spent many years gathering the brightest and best ideas, facts, and studies in order to provide the latest and most advanced answers and prognoses.

I struggled to devise a way to speak their language. I wanted to infuse them with the same enthusiasm I feel when sharing energy. Not everyone wanted a personal demonstration, so I needed to grab their interest by weaving words from their world.

I decided to discuss energy using the most basic sources.

From *Wikipedia.com* I found:
> Energy can be described as the capacity of a system to do work. In turn, work is defined as the result of application of a force through a physical distance (pushing a swing with a child in it ... carrying a bucket of water from the sink to the backyard). Due to the existence of a variety of forces in nature, energy and work have many different forms (gravitational, electric, heat, sound, etc.).
>
> Energy and its transformations (changes that occur); the direction of these transformations (coal burning causing electricity to be created), can vary from one natural science to another.
>
> In physics, energy is defined as the work of a certain force (gravitational energy causing the apple to fall).
>
> In chemistry, atoms and molecules, made up of electrically charged electrons and protons are rearranged (or moved) to create a change.
>
> In biology, growth, development and metabolism cannot be explained without invoking the energy concept. The sustenance of life itself is critically dependent on energy transformation (plants creating oxygen).
>
> Meteorological phenomena such as wind, rain, hail, lightening, tornados and hurricanes are all results of energy transformations brought about by solar energy (change).

Continental drift, mountain ranges, volcanoes, and earthquakes are phenomena that are a result of energy transformations in the Earth's crust.

Energy, an Introduction, by Anthony Carpi, Ph.D., 2003
Energy flows 'downhill' from a higher state to a lower one. For example, if a hot object and a cold object are placed next to each other, heat will flow from the hot object to the cold one ... a burning charcoal will cause an ice cube to melt.

From a Reiki standpoint, energy from a Universal source flows through a practitioner to a client, while 'used up', or 'older' energy moves from the client and returns to the Universe.

Thinkquest.org
Energy is a quantity associated with the state of a system. Energy can easily change forms and locations. Energy can be stored, conserved.

We should be able to track all the energy as it changes form, however there are forms of energy that are difficult, if not impossible for now, to count up.

We can still analyze a system that is being influenced by outside sources if we can describe how the outside forces are affecting the system.

Measuring energy transfer to a body from the Universal energy source can be a challenge. Because we have not discovered a consistently acceptable way to measure Reiki energy through one's hands does not mean that the energy does not exist.

After a Reiki session, a headache may have lessened, an insomniac may doze. Are these not a result or type of measure of Reiki energy?

Reality Check, The Energy Fields of Life
Victor J. Stenger, 1998
The unifying principle behind most alternative therapies is that some 'life force source' is responsible for infusing organisms with the property of life (energy).

A few centuries ago, the dualistic notion that soul or spirit or mind is an entity distinct from a materialistic world came into play. Spirit and body are expected to interact at some point. By influencing the spirit, perhaps the reaction can be traced to the body.

The concept of a special biological field within living things remains deeply engraved in human thinking. It is now working its way into modern health care systems, as now non-scientifically proven alternative therapies become increasingly popular.

A Practical Guide to Vibrational Medicine
Richard Gerber, MD, 2000
Vibrational energy includes sound waves, light, radio waves, television broadcasts, x-rays, cosmic rays, ultrasound waves and microwaves. Modern physics tells us that the only difference between these forms of energy is that each oscillates at a different frequency or rate of vibration.

According to the new perspective of Einsteinism and quantum physics, the biochemical molecules that make up the physical body are actually a form of vibrating energy.

The concept of the body as a complex energetic system is part of a worldview-gaining acceptance in the eyes of modern medicine.

Acupuncture is one form of "energy balancing." Reiki is another. Reiki therapy can recharge and rebalance the body's subtle energy patterns while relieving the effects of stress.

Chi gong supports the normal and balanced flow of ch'i energy.

Therapeutic massage is recognized in more and more hospitals and health centers as a stress reducing/health promoting 'hands on' technique.

Physical manipulation (chiropractic) applies a method of touching and manipulating the human body in order to create powerful restructuring, relaxing and healing effects.

The effect of touch upon human beings can be profound. Whether identified as psychological, energetic, or physical results, human touch can provide healing benefits on the physical body.

While these professional sources lay the groundwork for understanding energy, for some, Reiki has the mystical quality shared by those who believed the Earth to be round in the days that the flat concept was the norm. Because the idea may be beyond our day-to-day existence, how can it be? And yet, look at the many "ideas" that have come to be usual and normal—technical devices (I don't dare to call them phones) that connect us by voice, photo, text or internet, or laparoscopic surgeries that once included deep incisions, or tires that never go flat. Oh, wait, that is yet to come!

All I ask is that you open your mind and your heart and enjoy my stories, compare them to your experiences, and become aware of our connection.

Joy comes from using your potential.
—Will Schultz

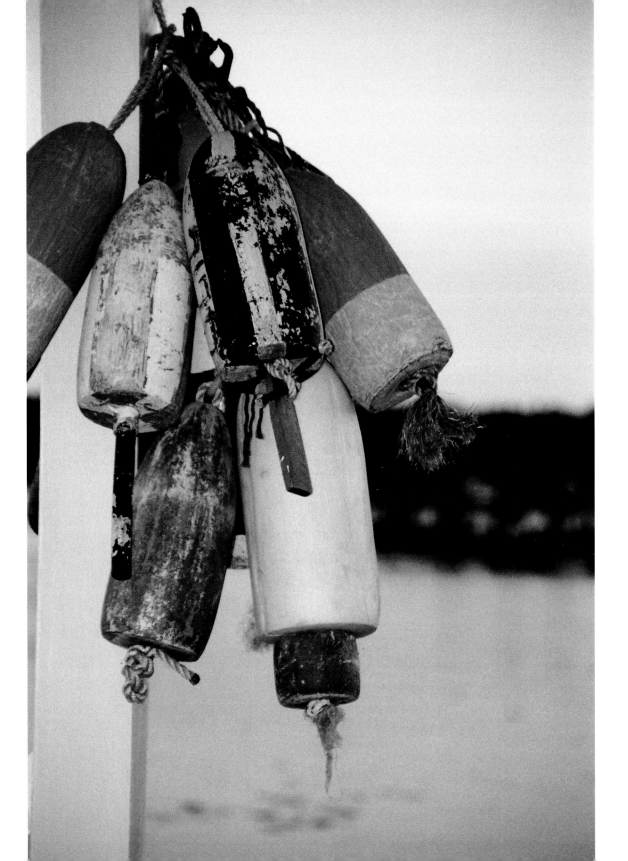

PASSING IT ON

A nursing home resident was referred to me after approval from his son. I am not sure how much the son knew about Integrative Therapy, but he wanted the best for his father. He visited him many times a week, but I never ran into him, nor did I hear his name. Whenever I reviewed the gentleman's care with a nurse, the son was always referred to as just that, his son.

My patient William was a dapper man. He always had a twinkle in his eye and a story to fill the afternoon. His reaction to Reiki was often to tell me a story from TV (his favorites were the old westerns) or to add a story about his past. He wove these tales into our afternoons of relaxation. William was happy to see me come and smiled with gratefulness as I left. He never complained and our relationship became a highpoint in my practice.

One day, William was in bed. He never dressed again. Television was no longer his pastime and his stories were finished. He quietly passed away after living a full, robust life.

I had planned to attend the visitation held in the chapel of the nursing home. I usually paid my respects in this way, even attending the funeral when appropriate. I suspected this visitation would be sparsely attended since the patient was quite elderly. I expected to add a presence to the room and anyway, I wanted to finally meet the son.

I arrived to discover that parking was a challenge. Something had been scheduled that drew in a large number of family and friends. I was delighted to discover that William's visitation was the attraction! Who would have guessed that this gentle soul would draw so many to pay their respects. As I made my way through the receiving line, I searched for the son, only to find daughters, granddaughters, grandsons and respective families, all calm and respectful, all thankful for my presence, all amazed that I had heard so many stories of their dad's or granddad's past. I also discovered that the twinkle in William's eye had been a lifelong enjoyment of the fair sex. He definitely had had a way with the ladies.

Within days, I learned why William's son had not been able to attend the visitation. He had been diagnosed with terminal cancer himself and was in the hospital at the time of his dad's passing. It was a reminder of life's hard twists. When he was discharged into hospice care, I volunteered to share Reiki with him.

I was surprised to realize I had known him during my career in banking. He was a larger than life presence within the community, the same position, I was to discover, that he also held within his family. Since I had never heard his name spoken, I never had made the connection. Although the family had not known of my visits to William in the nursing home, I gained the family's trust through Reiki, which was my gift to their husband, father, and grandfather, who was now getting ready for his own transition.

I normally offer Reiki to anyone and everyone around a patient, particularly the spouse. In this instance, his wife took these opportunities to remove herself from the vigil, and to lie down and drift away from the shocks of her day-to-day existence. The house sound system was always tuned to soft New Age music, a candle always available. Her oasis was wherever we found quiet and calm.

Theirs was a tightly knit family. I visited William's son until his death, and also shared Reiki with his sons, daughters, granddaughters, and friends.

Within hours of my last visit, he passed. The struggle was over. Another journey had begun for him as well as for the rest of the family. During our sessions, I had felt the strong bonds within the family and their close friends, and knew I had helped them all cope with the sudden departure of their leader, their anchor, their soul mate.

Over the following days and months, I heard many stories, saw many tears, and I joined in the laughter as memories were shared. I became "the Reiki lady" to anyone who came home, called, or sought me out. I became a friend to my patient's wife, and a support to her family. Today we continue to share stories, trials, and successes.

Just recently, William's great granddaughter flew home from her life at school to sort out her growing sorrows surrounding her grandfather's death. She happened to cross my path and we shared a few moments of Reiki. Afterwards she was able to return to her hectic days with a better perspective. Later she mentioned the effects of our meeting when chatting with her grandmother.

What began as a relationship with an elderly gentleman ending his days with westerns and memories, became one of friendship and caring for an entire family. I value this thread of connection and I acknowledge the gift of Reiki for bringing such a loving group into my life.

Joy is very infectious;
therefore, be always full of joy.
—Mother Teresa

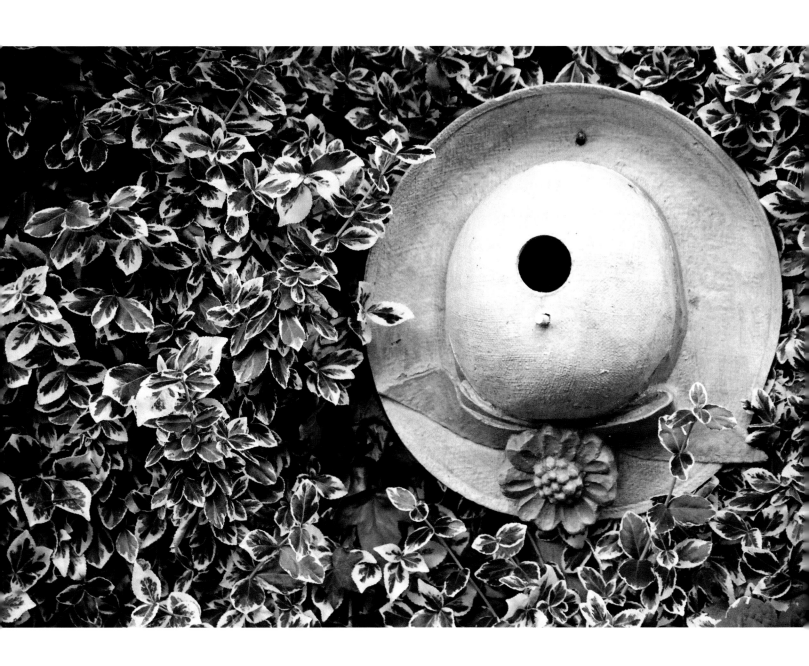

UNIQUE

I have always been a step out of line—a lightening rod for the uninspired plodders—a beacon in a professional group. I seem to travel through life pushing the envelope, choosing the road less traveled, branding all my activity with my own style, and dare I say, rules.

As I review the variety of career choices that I have made, one characteristic seems to weave its way through the winding path of my life: I seem to do everything under my terms and in my way. I have grown accustomed to succeeding by incorporating my brand on any traditional job.

My approach to Reiki is equally unusual—or is it? I was taught by a competent, loving soul. I scoured the examples of the "correct" hand positions. I kept a wristwatch by my client to make sure that the proper amount of time was spent in each approved hand position. I urged sharing experiences after each session.

I considered every step I made. Initially, I felt I needed a so-called treatment space in a professional building. That was the way to credibility. I made contact with a woman who was beginning a lease in a health-centered building. I was taken by surprise when she said she needed to "feel my energy" before

she would agree to share a space. I invited her to my home and we had a delightful conversation. I felt comfortable enough to share my questions about opening the Reiki energy—just what was the best procedure? She smiled—a smile I can only describe as Buddha-esque—and said, "It becomes natural and automatic as you gain experience." She continued to answer my naïve questions gently, but I didn't get it. I didn't understand that there is no right or wrong way to share Reiki.

There isn't just one way to share Reiki. There is no set of positions that must be followed. There is no time limit or required minimum. There is no specific result. There is no typical result. I acknowledge that my style and belief system may be a bit out of step with tradition, but I feel embraced by the non-judgmental blanket of Reiki.

There are different ways to describe the opening of your energy pathway— through attunement or initiation. Class size can vary from teacher to teacher. A single individual or a large group can constitute a class. Timing between classes can also be varied, again depending on the instructor. I have always believed that the right class of the right size with the most compatible teacher will present itself to the interested student at the right time.

Topics in each level of training seem to be varied, again much to my liking. I can start a Level 1 or 2 training with a particular agenda (my Virgo traits still rear up occasionally) and then smile as the topics discussed weave and change to the needs of the class.

Symbols, their use and the need for exact replication, create quite the discussion point within the Reiki community. Some take exception to sharing symbol drawing with non-attuned individuals, while others believe they are of no use unless the student is attuned to their use. Some practitioners never use the symbols after receiving them; some never share Reiki without using a complete set. You have to love the variety of beliefs.

Granted, I do believe a number of procedures are both suggested and needed to ensure respect for the power of Reiki, but even these I have found to be somewhat flexible, always keeping in mind the Reiki tenet that "Reiki does no harm." For instance, the need to share Reiki with a client who is lying down, or in a quiet space, is not totally necessary. I share

Reiki with a room of grieving individuals at a funeral; I gently place my hand on my friend's shoulder as she dodges tractor-trailers on the interstate; I am urged to place my hand on an anxious test-taking student's arm. Chaos swirling, only moments available, Reiki can affect anyone, at any time.

One-handed Reiki is acceptable. Sharing Reiki for thirty minutes in one position is effective. Sharing Reiki after a spicy dinner that included a glass of wine is allowed. Nothing is right or wrong. Reiki can do no harm.

Our unique, individual beliefs and styles all blend together as we join together to enhance energy's effect in our universe.

There is never a single approach
to something remembered.

—John Berger

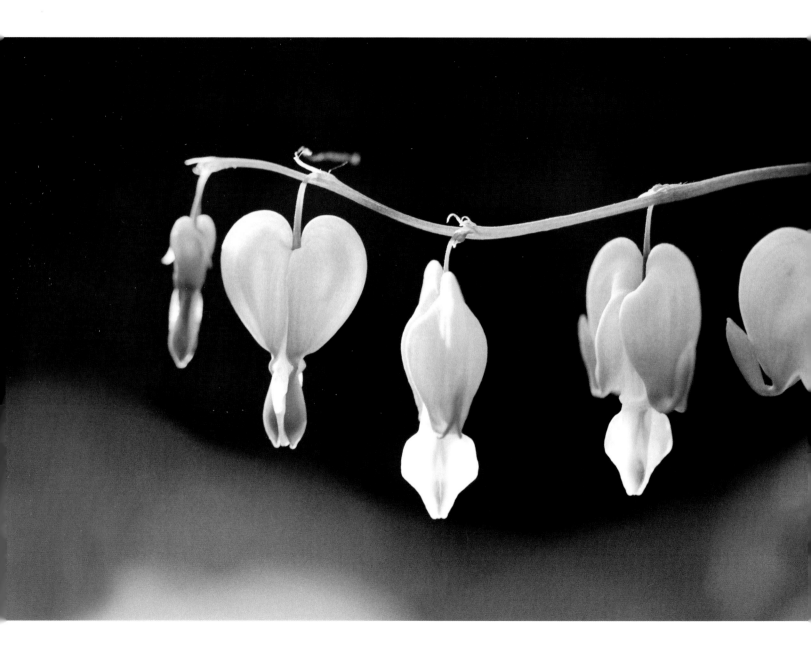

Valentine's Day is a celebration of love … an acknowl-edgment of feelings of caring and joy … a reminder to us of the beauty of demonstrating love.

This year, Valentine's Day included salutations from a variety of friends and loved ones. One well-wisher in particular is new to my sphere of influence, and we are in the process of getting to know one another. After a typical day of travel, he tends to check in and leave a message as he heads for home. On this par-ticular day, his wish was the hope that "I was with someone I love on Valentine's Day." I immediately gauged the "love" I had for the evening's planned companion … until I realized a whole new direction.

In a perfect world, we would always be with some-one we love … because we should love ourselves first and foremost! Don't we get urged to take care of ourselves first so we will be able to care for those around us? Isn't that the reason we are to put on the oxygen mask first? Don't we seek the ultimate in self-care in order to be the best we can be?

Self-Reiki can be the focus of that practice. With that intention, we receive the highest benefits of self-care. As we intend Reiki energy to fill us each day, we are able to feel and express our best. When we share Reiki in stressful situations, we know we will respond in the most appropriate manner possible.

If, however, we are part of the many who are so busy helping, caring, and sharing, that we lose sight of self, we may not be in the best condition to be of the greatest assistance. If we allow unkind emotions or thoughts to influence our day, we might have hurt-ful physical responses. If our energy is not running at its best, we may suffer the consequences.

As a latecomer to the need for self-Reiki, I ultimately realized the results of loving myself first. I continue to be drawn to Reiki to teach and share it with as many individuals as possible. My practice is extremely outward-driven, but I have seen my effectiveness increase remarkably as my use of self-Reiki has become a more regular part of my life.

As a test (because I am always testing), I have con-sciously spent time identifying moments that would be enhanced by self-Reiki. Obviously as I start (or finish) my day, I can take time to run Reiki through my body. It can be during a moment of thankfulness for another day, or during the contemplation of the day's events. It can include multiple hand positions, or a hand cradling a sore elbow. It can be consciously ended, or be completed naturally as I drift off to sleep. At these moments, I am thinking the best I can … about me! I actually love me! Well, you might say, those times are easy to set aside for the benefits of self-Reiki, but give me some ideas when real life intrudes! Crying babies, frustrated teens, irritated spouses, scheduled workmen…. All can jar our lives as we begin or end a day. It is up to us to take a moment to love ourselves with Reiki energy in order to handle those challenges.

Once we get out of bed, however, it can become a more conscious search for opportunities for self-Reiki. How about before (or during) a tense meeting, a doctor's appointment, a school conference, a rush hour drive, cooking a new recipe, caring for a parent … wait, how about any time during the day! The intention of helping our energy flow is the ultimate self-love action.

It is often said that we enter this world and leave this world alone. I believe that we enter and leave this world with the one we each love the most … ourself. It is only fitting that we should love the one we are with. Self-Reiki is a tool that will allow this desire to become a reality.

Sometimes your joy is the source of your smile, but sometimes your smile can be the source of your joy.

—Thich Nhat Hanh

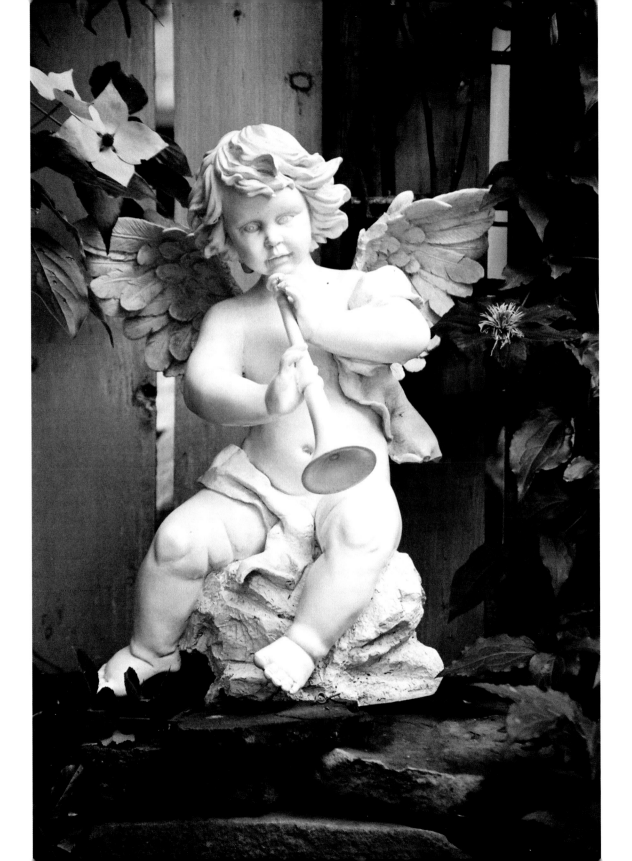

SEEING IS BELIEVING?

We live in such a literal world. Everyone wants proof, definitions, and facts. Left-brain is dominant for success ... mostly ... so far....

What we cannot "see" is not there, what we cannot measure does not exist. Why, if we believed such statements, science would close up shop and move on ... maybe to accounting. Even science butts heads with factions such as religion, logic, and politics.

Luckily, more and more, we are becoming aware that there just may be something to psychics, aura readers, medical intuitives, and the like. We might even admit that energy exists in many forms that we cannot see.

I met a chaplain once with a strong, gentle belief in God. She had an open mind and a beautiful spirit. Her left-brain had led her to success as the department head of pastoral care at a hospital, while her right brain had embraced Reiki. She was a student of mine who taught me much.

She was a cancer survivor when I met her. She had sparkle in her eyes and steel in her determination. As she advanced in her career, she gained respect and love. She was a private soul in her personal life, but she opened her heart to everyone. She had vision and passion. She had sweetness and joy.

Her cancer returned and spread. Her determination allowed her to finish projects and stay at the helm as long as she could without sharing her medical journey. Gradually her strength left her and she became homebound. I visited her often, offering her support, sharing, and Reiki. Although she struggled to remain calm in the eye of the cancer storm, eventually she was unable to continue to live alone and moved to a nursing home.

Such a nursing home! A personal suite of tastefully appointed areas allowed her visitors to carry on life's requirements and distractions. Some turned to needlepoint and knitting, others grabbed a hasty meal or dozed. Books, photo albums, and bibles were tucked around the tables and chairs. Few visitors were allowed into this sanctuary. The chaplain continued to protect her privacy as her vision slipped away and her pain increased. She became deliberate as she responded to all questions, even as the Inquisitor wandered.

I was one of the fortunate few who remained able to visit during these last days. My responsibility appeared to be to share Reiki ... and yet, I continued to bring a smile with my comments and observations. Often I feel that the smiles are as rewarding as the Reiki session. It became a challenge to coax a smile from her after a wisecrack left my lips.

Towards the end of her life, she commented on "others" surrounding her. Now this is not an unusual phenomenon, and we all know to go along with these sightings. I, of course, like to get specifics ... family? ... strangers? Just who are these protectors? I usually don't get a response, but I always try. The chaplain was no different. I never seemed to discover the identity of our fellow vigil keepers.

As she slipped from this life, those around her saw angels patiently supporting her journey. A peaceful calm enveloped the room. Her spirit moved from her body to travel with her angels.

Was I there? No. Did those in the room actually see the angels? Yes. Although the maxim is "seeing is believing," and even though I was not in attendance for her transition, do I believe angels were in the room? Yes.

Your life is a gift from the Creator.
Your gift back to the Creator
is what you do with your life.

—Billy Mills

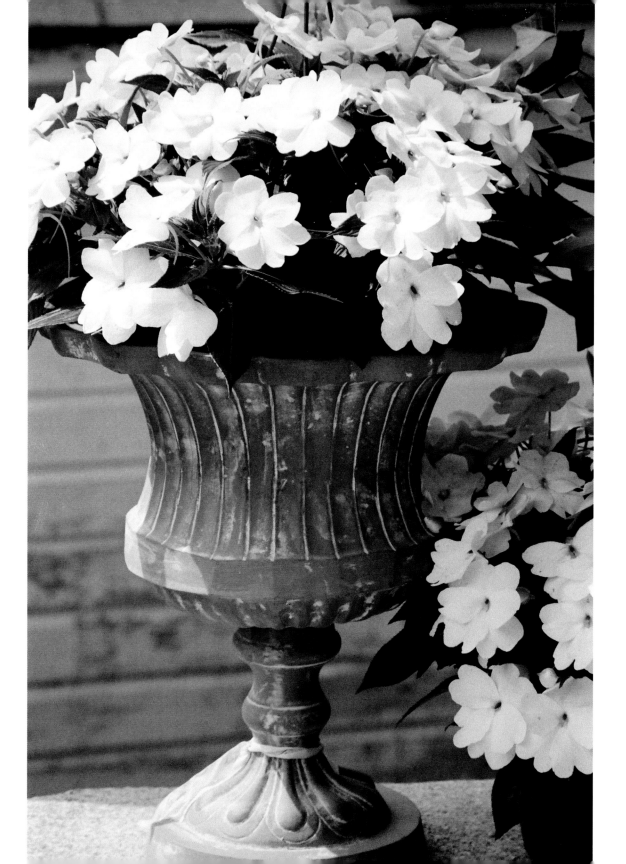

I have inherited many traits from my mother. This woman, the wife to a community leader, the mother of four, and active in her own right, had to learn tricks we all often need for survival and sanity. One trick that I learned from her was list-making.

I make lists (real and cerebral) for the day—sometimes by the hour. I have running lists for future shopping, lists for projects to accomplish (as if I would forget to rake the leaves swirling around my door), lists for thank you notes.

Making lists is one attempt to de-clutter the mind, to let niggling responsibilities be acknowledged and released from our minds at that moment. We can even make mental lists to support a stand we take in the debate of life.

For instance, I had a fairly substantial list of reasons for not having children. The list evolved over the years, beginning in my twenties and continuing for decades. Currently, I do not need a list as age has provided that brick wall. I have never regretted my choice, and my decision was validated when I experienced parenthood through stepchildren. Don't get me wrong. I enjoy children—step, young, older—but having my own was never a dream. But as a step-mom and an aunt, I have wonderful responsibilities and memories.

Likewise, I had a list of reasons (or rationalizations) for not attending funerals or visitations. I told myself that "I wanted to remember the deceased as a vital, joyful part of my life," that "I didn't want to add to the grief and tears experienced by the family during the long, grueling hours of visitation and funeral." In reality, I had no interest in standing over a dead friend and discussing how "lifelike he was." I had no ability to put into words what I thought the family could appreciate.

As I have experienced more death, and, as more dying has touched me, I have realized that my reasons for avoiding funerals were a bit selfish. A visitation, funeral, or celebration of life, can offer an opportunity to honor the deceased by sharing stories, saying a prayer, and smiling with love. What I perceived as a burden to the family is actually a chance to respect the life of the individual.

My response of choice used to be a simple card, sent shortly after the funeral, that included lofty sentiments and appropriate memories. Sometimes I pushed myself to attend a service or visitation, depending on my relationship to the survivors. I felt no need to be drawn into the line shuffling towards a group of Kleenex-holding strangers in order to say how sorry I was. But I did feel a hug was in order for a family with whom I had shared good times. That action usually elicited from me a quick story to gain a smile. I often felt drained and uncomfortable.

I can't say that the party after the ceremony was any easier. Granted, you had something to do (eat or drink, or often both). But those events often took on a jovial, disrespectful sheen that included commentary on who was doing what with or to whom. The family displayed a "deer in the headlights" demeanor and you had your fill of lasagna.

My awareness of others' needs expanded with my use of Reiki. I discovered that situations as well as people could be Reiki-ed. The calm introduced by Reiki energy can be utilized throughout a visitation, funeral, or any emotional farewell. I have offered Reiki during hospice memorial services as well as during visitations or funerals for individuals. I send Reiki to the energy generated in the gathering. As you are able to send Reiki by long distance to individuals, I send it throughout the room to help bring emotional peace to the individuals gathered there.

I have held my hand over the printed names of the recently deceased with the intention of sending Reiki to them in their new dimension. I have remained at a visitation and sent Reiki to the family standing in front of the casket. Reiki will relax the participants as if a calming hand has been placed on the shoulders of the mourners.

Individuals come to me after a memorial service to say they felt a peace come over them mid-service. I have seen a spouse move to a less emotional position in a receiving line at a visitation. I have watched a roomful of chatting funeral attendees take their seats and become quiet long before the beginning of the service. The emotional agitation often demonstrated by flitting around a funeral parlor can be calmed by Reiki.

I am now able to feel comfortable at a visitation or funeral. Giving myself Reiki before the event allows my energy to be at its best. Reiki has given me a way to comfort a grieving family or friends. I now can attend these events, offer my support, and provide a calming effect during an emotional transition in life.

Most importantly, I now can tear up my list for not attending funerals.

Maybe now is the time to evaluate my list of reasons for not exercising....

Grief can take care of itself, but to get the full value of joy you must have somebody to divide it with.
— Mark Twain

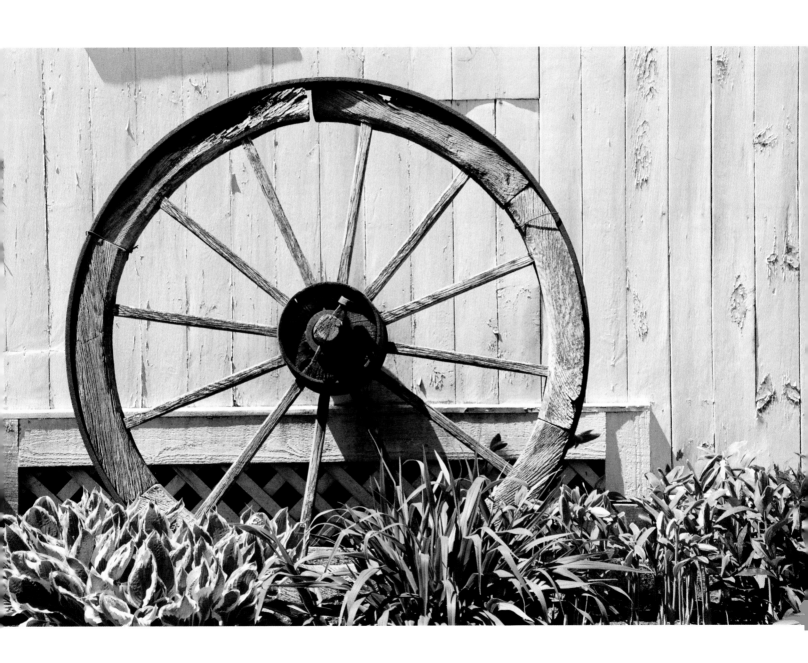

AT A DISTANCE

Many a prayer and wish have been sent through the cosmos. From time to time, each of us has wished to be geographically nearer to a loved one in time of need or crisis in order to provide support, calm, or touch. Whether it is a relative or a friend who is in the hospital or suffering from emotional trauma or facing a daunting meeting or other stress situation, we choose how to offer our energy.

For those who believe that any thought is an action, and, as a result, has a corresponding reaction, then long distance Reiki is not a stretch. Documented results of prayer, evidence of thoughts becoming real, and the proven power of intention all support the theory that energy can be sent to another location. Long distance Reiki is practiced in a variety of forms with a number of procedures. It can be a few moments of intention or an hour of organized meditation.

It was perhaps the most difficult for me to incorporate into my practice. After being trained to perform this Reiki, I would set a pre-determined time with my recipient, light candles, play music, and hold a picture or place my hands on an imaginary head. As I shared Reiki, I would envision specific hand placements and move around the body. I used long distance

Reiki almost exclusively for the medically ill or surgery-bound patient. In my eagerness for results, I would call my client after the session to obtain a report. A bit rigid you might say, but at that point I still needed validation.

But then real life knocked on my door. The son of a dear friend was sitting for a state bar exam. She asked me to join her in sending energy to him for the days of the test. I eagerly set the stage. We selected a favorite place of her son's to meet. It was summer and the outdoors beckoned. In fact, we sat at a picnic table shaded by trees, surrounded by thick grass. This location included an icy treat stand, and the owner took note of us—probably because he was not yet open and we looked as if we were anticipating a waitress, bustling over to fill our order. When we explained our intentions to the owner, he provided cups of flavored ice, Jimmy Buffet music, and his best wishes.

Instead of candles, music, or photos, we sat and shared experiences about her son and his life's journey to this point. We envisioned him in the classroom, what he had on, how he held his pencil, studied his posture. We laughed and sighed over the humorous and exciting memories. During this exchange of thoughts, I was sending long distance Reiki. Each of us provided love and intention in our own way.

One of the highest held beliefs in the practice of Reiki is that Reiki heals rather than cures. So in this situation, I was sending Reiki for her son to be the best he could be during the exam rather than asking for him to ace the test. We wanted him to answer as many questions correctly as possible, sure, but I wanted Reiki to calm him, focus him, keep him in the moment, not necessarily to guide his pencil to the correct answers. Reiki would help diminish anxiety, reduce leg jiggling, keep eyes clear, acknowledge time limits, hide hunger pangs, and whatever else might interfere with test-taking. This long distance Reiki was sent with love and respect. It was sent without the knowledge of what the outcome of the exam would be, or how the outcome would fit into the mosaic of his life.

He made contact after the testing concluded and his relief was evident. He appreciated the energy, in whatever form that it had been shared. We do not need defined results in order to gauge the usefulness of energy that is shared with love. We do not need medical trauma to see the effectiveness of Reiki.

As a postscript to this example, my friend's son did not pass the exam on his first try. He went on to use a tutor and sailed through on his next attempt. His path included disappointment. Perhaps this disappointment shifted his work ethic, perhaps not everything would come so easily to this young man. Perhaps the second attempt made him a better attorney. And with this outcome, Reiki made him the best he could be.

One joy scatters a hundred griefs.
—Chinese Proverb

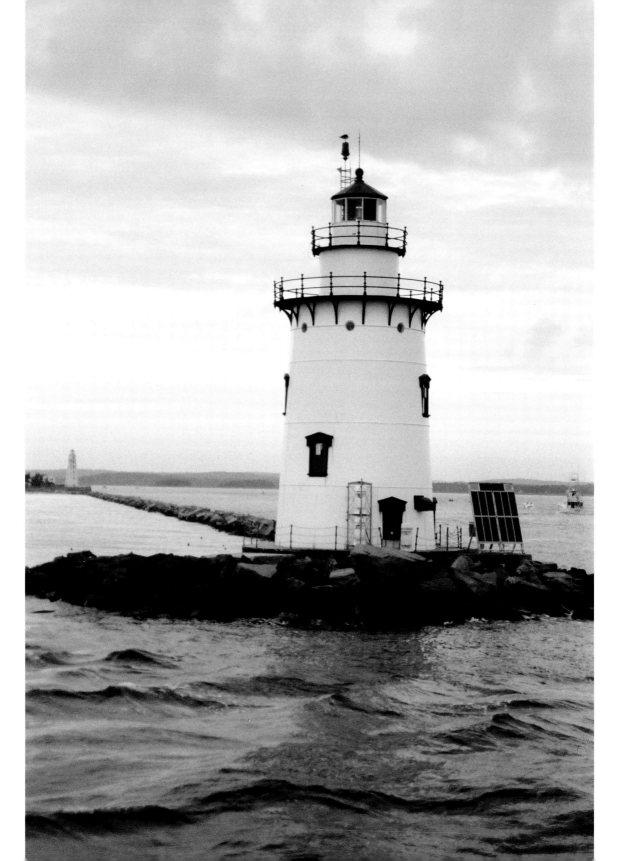

LOSING CONTROL

I have a client who reminds me of my grandmother. My maternal grandmother is a legend in our family. As a young widow with two small children, she went back to school for an advanced degree and never looked back. She held prestigious positions from New England to Arizona and managed to sail the seas and whitewater raft well past retirement age. In fact, she retired numerous times! She finally remarried at the age of eighty-four—to a man she had known in high school—and enjoyed more than ten active years of married life before she became a widow yet again. Grandmother Hazel lived past her one-hundredth birthday, and her spirit has never left our family.

My grandmother's strongest trait was her seemingly impenetrable control over her life, the circumstances surrounding her, and her loved ones. To those of us who admired her, her invisible hold over everyone and everything was awe-inspiring.

We humans seem to strive for control. Whether it is control over ourselves, our lives, or of others, we feel a sense of power when we think we are in control. For most of our lives, this illusion propels us down our life paths. It is often at life's end that we discover this "control" issue holds us back from moving forward.

My client Lucille can claim a cornucopia of accolades. She is a well educated, well traveled ninety-seven-year-old lady. She has won numerous awards for her tireless efforts with nonprofit organizations. She raised five successful, well adjusted children almost single-handedly (her husband traveled extensively). She bungee jumped at the same age that my grandmother rode the Colorado Rapids.

Sadly, Lucille is dying. She received a terminal prognosis over a year ago. She had stubbornly refused to believe that prognosis. In fact, I would say, she had exerted her legendary control over her situation and hadn't entertained the thought of death, or discussed her future with her family.

I was referred to Lucille and her family when medical professionals feared the end was near. That was over six months ago. I watched this proud lady as she continued her control over her family and her surroundings, and then I watched her frustration and anger as her control began to slip away.

Reiki helps soothe our emotions by "relaxing" our essence into a calm awareness. It allows us to let go of behaviors that are shields that might hide our true issues.

Reiki is often suggested as a tool to work in tandem with counseling. When combined, a treatment plan can be swifter and more successful. It is as if the body relaxes into awareness and the client can work through whatever layers of problems that might exist.

Losing control is a frightening thought. At the end of life, every control we have held dear is stripped away. Our freedom, our minds, our spirits slip away. Reiki allows us to accept our destiny with understanding and joy.

Lucille (who, by the way, still doubts Reiki's effectiveness, but enjoys our conversations) has begun the end of her life's journey. She has lost control over her surroundings, her family, and at times, her body. Her mobility has been compromised and she has become frustrated. And yet, I am seeing her gradually let go. She is starting to talk about dying and death. She is making every goodbye more meaningful. She is vocalizing her love for those around her more often. She accepts my kisses with smiles instead of showing irritation.

Reiki has supported Lucille's transition into awareness. She now dozes instead of argues. She reminisces easily and proudly. She is more content. She has opened her spirit to the exciting adventure ahead. She is preparing. She is giving up control.

Joy is a net of love by which you can catch souls.
A joyful heart is the inevitable result
of a heart burning with love.

—Mother Theresa

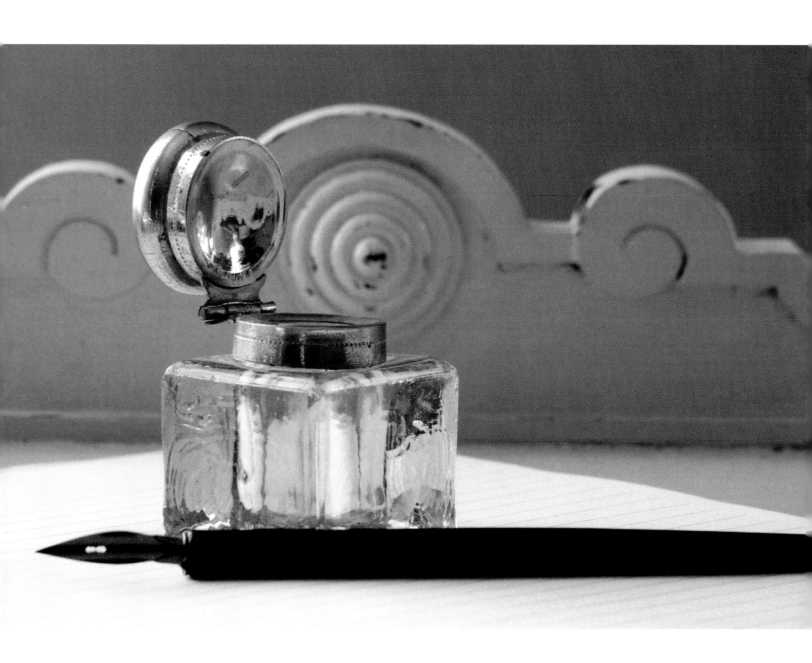

THE NUDGE

Creative writing, whether fact or fiction, can be a work of art that brings joy to many. Creative writing can heal, educate, humor, and challenge its readers. It is with great humility that most authors approach the task of sharing the written word. Although I have repeatedly been urged to write by psychics and astrologers alike, I always felt that I used my communication skills in a more professional capacity, for training and negotiating, and to tell a joke or two!

I never saw myself as an author. I don't see myself as an author even now. I see myself as a teacher with stuff to say. I see myself as someone who desires to share experience and belief with as many people as possible. I don't believe I have the answers, the true path, or the way. I have a passion that has propelled me down one path of this maze, which I call my life, and this is the path I wish to share. As a result, I am an author.

So, as an author, I find myself falling into the traditional "artist procrastination" trap. I can give you a pile of reasons for not writing that would fill a book ... maybe my second book? I have been using those many and varied reasons for the last few months. "The weather is too nice ... or too bad." (That multi-purpose excuse also has worked well for any exercise plan I try to implement.) "I have too much to do." But what can be more important than sharing my passion, you ask? Although I resist structure, I have been successfully employed for years. See what I mean?

Then yesterday, it all fell into place ... and fall is the operative word. A close friend and I are doing a study on tacos in town. The best meat, spices, cheese, shell, size ... a study that is of value only to two taco-loving best friends. As we approached the door to the latest contestant (we are probably half way through our list), I tripped over a handicapped ramp at the front door and went sprawling across the concrete. This body does not fall gracefully or well. My head "bounced" (according to my friend), my glasses cut into my face, and my watch shattered. My body probably screamed in agony at every contact it made with the concrete. (Did I already mention that exercise is not my friend?)

The blood dripping from my face led bystanders to believe I was in a bad way while I was mostly concerned about ruining a beloved scarf. Anyway, enough about the fall. I just want you to understand the condition I was in when I finally returned home. (As an aside, blood gives you priority and excellent care in any "doc-in-a-box.")

I returned home with stitches, facial scrapes, a jammed pinky that did not allow me to sign emergency forms with ease, and potential dual knee issues—not to mention my weak back, which always reminds me of my limitations whenever jarred, exercised, or abused. All this and I never even had the pleasure of a taco!

The afternoon progressed as an array of friends discovered my plight, both energy workers and "straights" alike. I spent a big part of the remainder of the day taking calls from concerned friends and then taking re-calls from the same friends into the evening. Since I decided to lay low, my otherwise hectic schedule came to an abrupt halt. The only exhaustion I faced was a sore phone ear.

During those hours, I gave myself Reiki ... while on the phone, watching TV, and otherwise twiddling my thumbs. My energy friends sent Reiki as well. Although I did not ask, I am confident that each friend sent love, prayers, or energy ... whichever tool they use to assist others.

Now, this is where it gets wild. I went to bed with my face smeared in anti-bacterial cream, instead of the latest anti-aging concoction. I blessed my body for taking care of me, but allowed for the ugly face, stiff knees, and achy back that might greet me in the morning.

I awoke after a fairly decent sleep. I gingerly got out of bed—to a body without aches! I checked my face and the angry red scrapes had significantly faded and the anticipated bruising was not there. Yes, I did look as if something had happened—after all, stitches equate to drama. I calmly told anyone viewing the damage that I was in the process of a facelift, and that I was doing

this one eye at a time. (I hate to report that some might have taken this tidbit as truth.)

I firmly believe that Reiki changed the outcome of my fall. My body was the best it could be. I was amazed that I felt great. No excessive bruising. In fact, no bruising on the knees that had attempted to keep me away from the concrete. My pinky worked fine. My back just twinged a bit ... maybe no worse than a day on my feet. My face was not red at the site of the scrapes.

My friends and I used Reiki to "heal" this mature body, and in doing so, nudged me to return to writing. Thank you.

Such is human psychology
that if we don't express our joy,
we soon cease to feel it.

—Lin Yutang

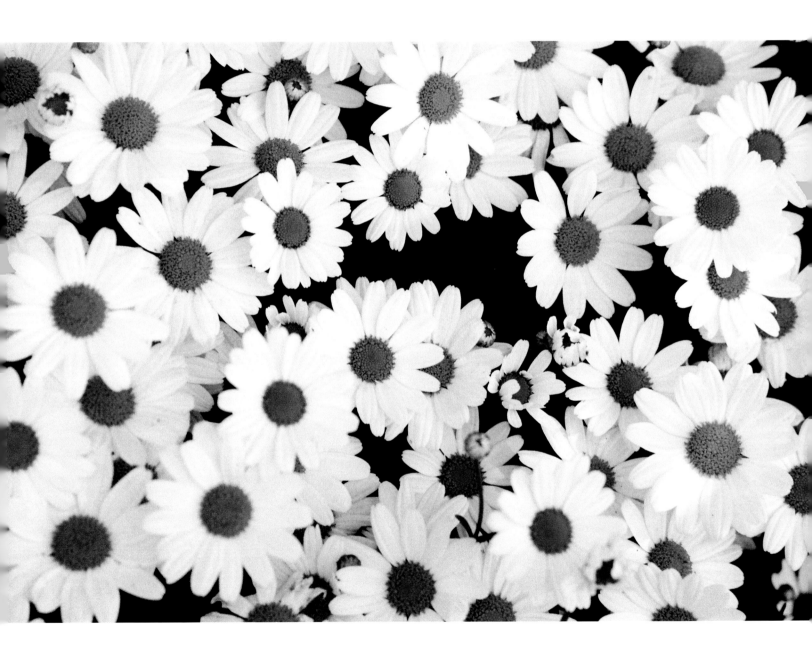

WARM AND FUZZY

I love the term "warm and fuzzy." I love how it makes me feel. I love how I can feel it even in the hot, humid days of summer. That leads to the question of what "warm and fuzzy" means to me. It describes security, sweetness, and contentment to me. I am sure it was originally connected to the first teddy bear (or soft dog, in my case) and the joy it gave me. Many sights, sounds and tastes take me to "warm and fuzzy." Better yet, it leads to an enormous pot of feelings.

This umbrella of feelings can encompass as diverse a group of emotions as there are types of umbrellas! Understanding feelings, communicating feelings, comparing feelings—whew! Sometimes the mind boggles at the thought of knocking at the door to our feelings. What may be warm and fuzzy to me, may illicit a blank stare from another.

Just as we each have individual sets of feelings, we each have unique ways of "feeling" energy. As we become aware of the unlimited potential of sharing energy, we open ourselves to the variety of ways of feeling the experience.

Traditionally, when sharing Reiki, we sense energy through hand heat, hand sensing cool, hand tingling—

all ways of determining energy movement, the lack of movement, or shifts in it. Practitioners' hands can vibrate, rock, or massage as they send energy to the client. Even fingers, as hand extensions, can shoot energy from their tips. Hands are the well-known symbol of energy transfer.

I have a student who smells the heat of energy as he practices. He describes it as the smell of the sun hitting your body as you bask on the beach. (Well, I am not sure he actually said "on the beach," but that adds a great visual.) You know that smell ... an iron ready to press a shirt, the electric range burner that you accidentally turn on that isn't under your saucepan.... Those are the smells of heat.

I never thought that other parts of the body could feel energy, but our sense of smell "feels" by odor, right? I know another practitioner who has "heard" the pulsating energy move through a client's body and has heard the static of partially blocked energy struggling to move. Ears and energy. What a unique feeling.

Visual feelings of energy are many and varied. A number of practitioners see guides, angels, or loved ones as they work on clients. These supporting characters could be there for the client or the practitioner. Regardless whom they are there for, the resulting feeling is love. Isn't "Help is all around us." a key saying?

At times, snapshots, which explain, remind, or question, are splashed behind our closed eyes. I have seen unrecognizable people who later are explained to me by the client's surprising revelations.

The color and the feelings experienced by a practitioner during a session are visual clues to energetic activity. Often we translate color to chakra activity and can feel the abundance or lack thereof, whichever might be appropriate. Color denotes feelings in a broad range of emotions such as creation, growth, or spirit.

As we calm, soothe, release, clear, and support with Reiki, we are able to identify and experience a variety of feelings. Both practitioner and client are able to feel with all their senses. Often what is experienced by the practitioner is not related to the reported feelings of the client. This is what is special and unique. All of these feelings allow each of us to interpret our experiences in our own way, with our own feelings.

We are all looking for "warm and fuzzy."

Joy is the feeling of grinning on the inside.
—Melba Colgrove

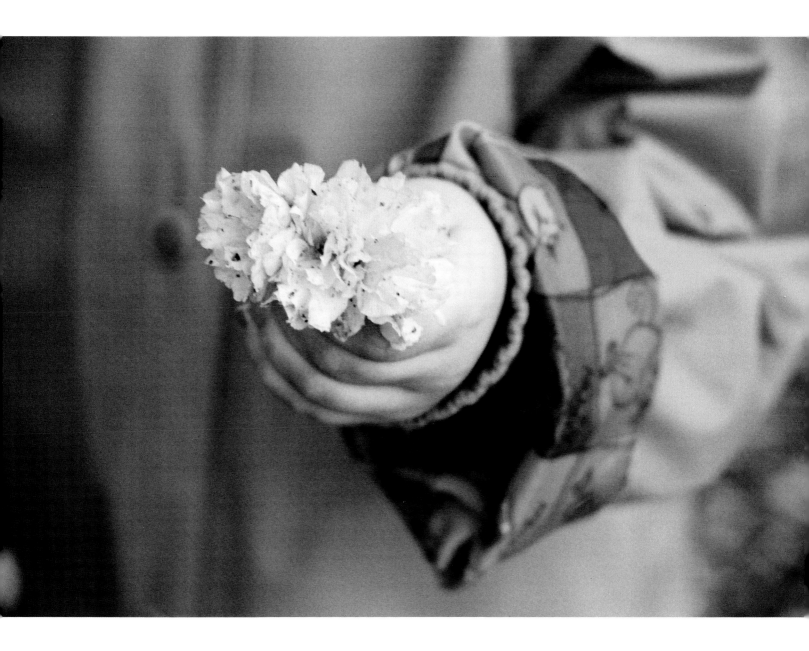

FROM THE MOUTHS OF BABES

As my mother reached the Autumn of her full life, she gave her family and friends many gifts. Gifts, such as determining on her own when to end her driving career, were given to us and made our relationship that much smoother. She had the strength and awareness to let go of activities that could complicate an aging lifestyle.

So, when she believed she would be safer if she had assistance with showering, it fell to me to find that special person who would be strong enough to aid a larger woman, and who would also have a personality that my mom would enjoy. After mentioning my need to various friends, I was given a name of a lady who had an errand-running service. It was up to me to discover if she would take on a bathing client.

Edyth became an indispensable member of our team, which included family and friends. She gradually became a member of our family, and to this day, offers the same calming influence to those around her that she gave to my mother, all the while maneuvering through her own path of challenge. Edyth, a retired public administrator, has become the caregiver to five of her grandchildren. Now, I don't know about you, but when I retire, taking on another family would not

be my choice for relaxation. Not so for Edyth! She glows as she recites the accomplishments of each child in sporting events, choir performances, and school activities.

Just after my first attunement, Edyth urged me to share Reiki with her oldest granddaughter. This seven-year-old was having trouble sleeping and Edyth thought the calming effect of Reiki energy might help her nightly struggles. She also mentioned that this young lady had a natural gift for massage.... Her hands were soothing and strong.

Since she would be my first child client, I was not prepared for the immediate reaction that I have since encountered with almost all my young clients—she fell asleep soon after I placed my hands on her. I was astonished that a person who had sleeping issues could zonk out on a massage table in someone else's home. I was gratified that, upon waking, Edyth's granddaughter said she "liked that just fine." Only one visit, but it was a milestone for both of us. Gradually, the sleeping crisis passed and Edyth repeatedly said she wished her granddaughter could learn Reiki. As I was just beginning my own Reiki journey, I was not equipped to teach, and I had to decline the request.

Fast-forward several years. I had moved out of state and had become a Reiki Master/Teacher. I returned to my hometown to continue my practice and Edyth remained part of my life. She again mentioned teaching her granddaughter. Although I have had a number of children as clients, this would be my first child student. Being the explorer that I am, I did not hesitate to agree. I knew that Edyth was too overwhelmed with day-to-day life for her to bring Reiki into her family successfully. Yet, here was a chance to introduce this energy into a family that cried for soothing calm. Here was a student who could slow the pace of her siblings, relax her grandmother, and help in the emotional drama of a growing family.

As I studied and researched teaching Reiki to a child, I discovered the challenges that would be present in her path. I carefully re-wrote my class book and made it relevant to a teen.... After all, what eleven-year-old in today's world wants to be reminded of not even having attained teendom!

Around adults, Edyth's granddaughter charms and quietly demonstrates an awareness beyond her years. Could she be one of those called "an old soul?" She was eager and attentive ... well, until I caught a yawn and discovered that we had been talking non-stop for over two hours without a break. I don't even suggest that for my adult students!

We spent the day figuring out opportunities for sharing Reiki with her family. We discussed the importance of respect for privacy, and the joy of relaxation. We even discussed her use of healing touch instead of the more aggressive shoving and hitting of peers. I love the one-on-one teaching approach, particularly with the young or the shy. They open up to the energy with un-abashed excitement. It was a special day for both of us.

Part of my typical class includes an energy session with me, the teacher. Whether that comes during the inter-view process before the class date, or during class, it is my gift to the student. Edyth's granddaughter eagerly began her personal Reiki session. We had most of the classroom work behind us, and, because we had shared Reiki years ago, I knew she was aware of the elements of hands-on Reiki. Again, she slipped almost immedi-ately into sleep, a slight snore competing with the soft music. It is always an awesome privilege to connect with another person. I believe that we both are honored.

Upon the conclusion of the session, I gently woke her by removing her eye pillow. I always give a client some re-adjustment time, but before I left the room, she smiled, looked right into my eyes, and said, "It feels so good."

As with all children, the feeling that I was useful was perhaps the greatest joy I experienced.
—Eleanor Roosevelt

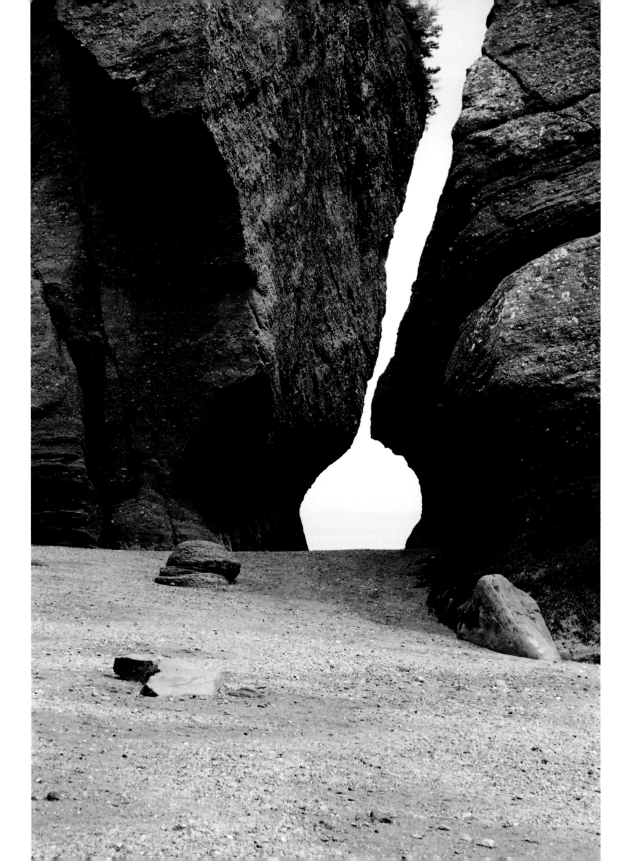

BEFORE AND AFTER

One of the most rewarding opportunities to share Reiki occurs pre- and post-surgery. Whether the surgery is planned or is an emergency, Reiki is the perfect tool to prepare the body for a change.

When I first became involved with energy healing, I encountered the option of preparing the body for surgery by "talking" to that part of the body, which was to be operated upon. For instance, "discussing" your upcoming hysterectomy with your abdominal area was urged. Not only would you explain the surgery to your affected area, but you would also thank the organ to be removed for its help over the years. By blessing the event, the fear lessens. The knowledge that comes from reviewing the surgical procedure can calm the cellular structures involved.

When first presented with this concept, I raised my eyebrow in doubt. "Talk to the uterus? Thank it for all that cramping and bleeding?" But then I realized that many, if not most, uteri were wondrous homes to babies and the center of a woman's femininity. Many women would mourn the loss of their wombs and by doing so, possibly affect the surgery and the healing process.

I took this concept further and reviewed all types of surgery. Whether removing an organ, excising a tumor, setting broken bones, or replacing a hip, why not take a mental inventory of the procedure? Why not review the fun that hip has had over the years? And, for that matter, why not discuss with your tumor why it needs to go? In doing so, your thoughts become actions, actions that release fear through information, all the while soothing and thanking a nervous gall bladder.

Upon introducing this idea to a client, explanation is key to his participation. I often compare this to meditation or prayer—with a bit more kick or focus! I sometimes include a guided meditation as a suggestion for the path of his thoughts—something like "Let's thank your lung for the terrific job it has done keeping you filled with oxygen all these years. Every breath in and out is a miracle of bringing in life's sustenance and removing toxins. You might tell the skin, fat (yes, there is probably that), and muscles in the chest area that there will be some disruption soon, as a knife, laparoscope, or other invasive tool will be entering and interrupting their perfect vibrations. You might say you are preparing them for the surgery. Then, quietly discuss the procedure with your body ... always softly and calmly, either out loud or in your mind."

After surgery, in fact, I urge upon waking in recovery that the client immediately thank his body for doing such a great job getting through the procedure! A message of calm and relief to the surgical site promotes the healing.

So, where's the Reiki? All this goes on while Reiki is being given. As the energy promotes the free flowing balance of vibrations, the client's thoughts act as guides and points of joy.

I usually discuss the number of visits that the client feels comfortable with, both pre- and post-surgery. This plan varies from client to client. I do not push a particular schedule for my visits, unless asked for input. Experienced Reiki practitioners may offer various packages, and each may be different and yet perfect for that client. Again, nothing is structured. I have had clients who wanted 3 or 4 sessions before surgery while some only feel one session is necessary. Post-surgery is similar with the client calling the shots. I am often outside the recovery area giving long distance Reiki. I have been called to hospital rooms; I have been called for a session days after the recovery has begun. I have learned to be gently available.

Many clients report significant differences in surgery or other medical procedures if Reiki is involved. The client may be calmer, awaken faster and clearer from the anesthesia, or experience less pain. He may heal at the surgical site more quickly than in the past, or than the average patient. Nausea is lessened when Reiki is included in a treatment plan. The client may recuperate faster, may have less fear or anger, and may remain calmer during the healing process.

Reiki will allow the client to be the best patient he can be.

The joy of a spirit is the measure of its power.
—Ninon de Lenclos

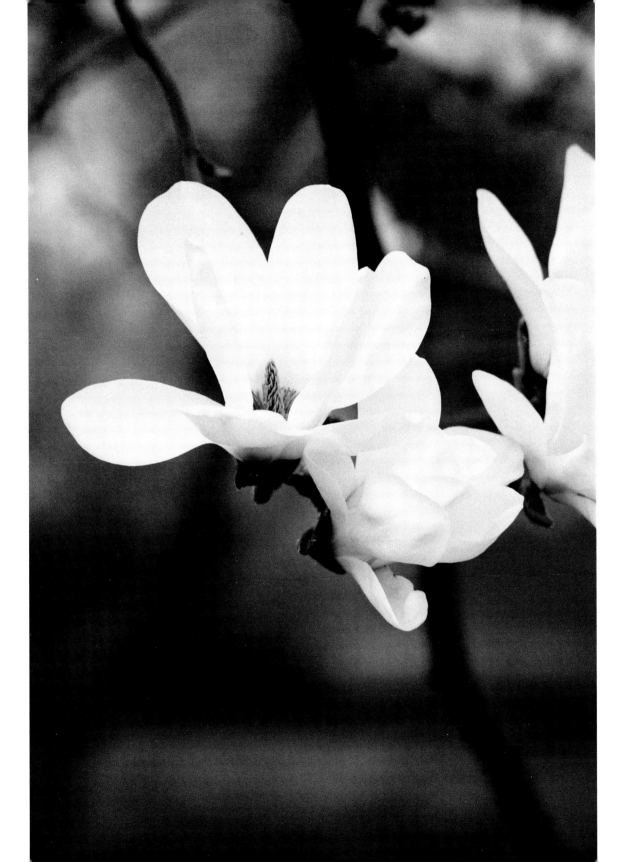

THE KISS

Alzheimer's is a slippery slope, and slope is the perfect word for the downward spiral one's mind takes when affected by this devastating disease. Reaching a diagnosis, accepting the course the disease will take, and suffering the results are experiences shared by the patient and his loved ones. Even the medical professionals feel the frustration and despair.

I have been honored to work with an Alzheimer's unit of care, one well known in our community. The number of patients varies, but the average number of residents hovers around twenty, all in various stages of Alzheimer's. Some chat, wander, participate; others sleep, stare, and cry. All of these patients are loved, nurtured, and cared for by a group of special people. I always see smiles, patience, and support. Laughter is encouraged, and humor is welcome.

Confusion is dealt with daily. Residents wonder what time it is, what their names are, who is bathing them, where were they born, and what has happened to their pasts. Caregivers respond with calm, loving answers, often non-answers, that appear to satisfy the immediate need to know. There are those who never question and rarely answer, but at times, do seem aware of the love surrounding them.

Although I love to chat with the more verbal patients, I treasure those who have slipped away to another place, a place that has removed them from the alert status needed to function in today's world. These souls spend much of their time sleeping and are roused to dress, eat, or visit with family or medical staff. No questions are asked and no memories are made.

Reiki is a perfect gift for the Alzheimer's patient. Confusion can lessen, anxiety diminish, and sleep deepen. I know my client is the best he can be after a session of Reiki. Although I always receive permission from the family to share Reiki with a resident, I still ask for permission from the patient. I know the client may not understand my question, but I trust our higher selves to sort that out. There have been times when a patient sensed the energy and pulled away. On those occasions I cease sharing, remove my hands, wait a moment, and start again, without touch. If I detect withdrawal again, I know I am to share time but not Reiki on this visit. I have no feelings of failure or lack of ability. I know today I am to sit quietly or in a low, one-sided conversation.

I had a special resident who usually slept quietly during Reiki sessions. Lily was a petite, fairy-esque lady, always curled up with her stuffed animals or a decorated pillow. Her hair was lovingly gathered atop her head with a ribbon or clasp that matched the colors she wore that day. Lily was a favorite, and everyone allowed her moments of yelling or frowning when she was irritated or hurting. Reiki allowed her to gently snore, un-tense her curled body, and otherwise calm her limited existence.

Occasionally Lily woke up. (I usually remain away from a sleeping patient's head so that no one is startled upon waking.) She sometimes opened her eyes and gazed at my face. I always explained, in a basic fashion that would slide over her mind, who I was and what I was doing. One time she grabbed the photo badge hanging around my neck, studied it and smiled. I like to think she enjoyed my picture.

An event that touched my heart took place during what began as an uneventful visit. Old big band songs were drifting over residents in the gathering room as medical staff was bustling around with medications and cookies, quietly murmuring greetings and comments. Lily was snoozing on the cloud of caring that supported her. My hands were placed on her elbow and in her hand. She opened her eyes, gazed at me,

brought my hand to her lips and gently kissed it. I knew she was thanking me for her feelings of peace. I knew she was acknowledging the joy she experienced with Reiki. I am sure she saw my eyes light with gratitude and love.

To have joy one must share it.
Happiness was born a twin.

— Lord Byron

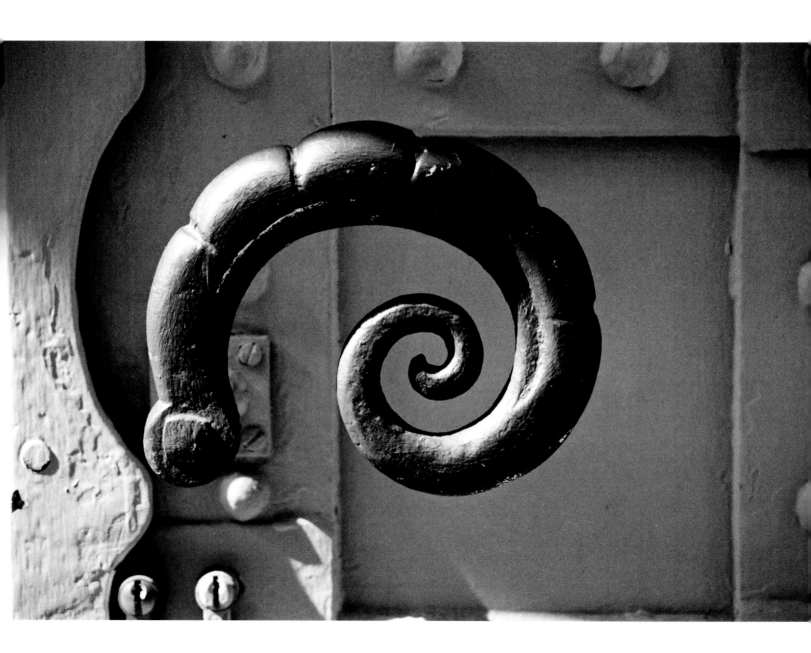

WHO'S IN CHARGE HERE?

As youngsters, many of us are urged to be independent, self-sufficient, and accomplished. We are measured and shaped. If we are "successful," wc have become the engineer of our train, the wind beneath our own wings. We learn that we are "in charge" of our destiny.

Interestingly enough, at some point, we each also may have become aware of a superior power, force, or being, depending upon our belief systems, which may open or even direct our individual paths. This potential influence may weave itself into the fabric of our lives, bringing us either support and peace, or more turns and more questions.

As we recognize this possibility, we have a dilemma. After all the talk about being strong, powerful, and independent, how does something or someone else take charge or know more?

We are functioning participants in this thing we call life, and we pride ourselves on a certain amount of control in order to be independent, self-sufficient, and accomplished. We employ our minds and hearts to structure whatever controls we feel we need to keep ourselves on our chosen paths. Choosing what clothes to wear, how to speak coherently, whether to follow a religion, how to be gainfully employed … these are just a few of the controls we place in our lives.

Although control can be used on the path to accomplishment, we often unnecessarily attempt to control our loved ones, our environment, and our futures. In fact, control can become a detriment to our enlightenment (did I actually use that word?). Control can become a negative force in our lives if we allow it to reign.

It is human nature, well, it is my human nature to attempt to control my environment and, to some extent, my future. When I began my Reiki path, I felt that my environment affcctcd my abilities to share Reiki. I created a soft, calm, healing room with low lights, candles burning, and music playing softly. I just knew the energy flowed much stronger in the correct environment.

At the same time, I needed to know what was going on in my client's body and life. I often felt I needed to "direct" the flow of Reiki to particular parts of the body. I would "talk" to the energy and tell it where to go and what to do! I thrived on discovering the needs of my client (emotional and/or medical) and then "zapping" that part of the body that I thought was affected. As I placed my hands on the prescribed area of the body, I "directed" the energy to smooth out the static created by the "dis-ease." I was shoving energy around to my specifications, as if the energy were in my control.

Is anyone laughing yet?

When we have the honor of sharing Reiki with a person in pain (physically or emotionally), who are we to know immediately what the cause of that pain might be? Or how should we know just what will occur as Reiki energy floods that person? I have spent moments hovering over an individual's heart in an attempt to improve blood flow or remove emotional blocks, thinking all the while that I had all the answers and control. What would you say if those specific heart problems originated because of major issues with the client's security or survival beliefs? Why would I not focus, then, on the First Chakra located at the base of the body's trunk where these issues have been identified to lie? What sort of "control" did I demonstrate?

Reiki energy knows where to go and what to do in order for us to be the best we can be. We as practitioners need not know all the aches and pains (physical and/or emotional) before we begin sharing Reiki. We really only need to know if the client is comfortable and accepting of potential hand placement. We really only need to keep our hearts open for intuitive direction. If we allow our "control" to interfere, we are only adding static to the atmosphere. We are not listening as we might. We are not keeping our "straw" clean and open for energy to flow easily to the client. Now that I mention this, I must say that I have found that our attempts to "control" almost anything usually only add unneeded complications or static to our lives!

I remember early Reiki sessions, when, in my desire to help, I asked, "What hurts?" If someone complained of arthritis pain in the knee, that became my focus. After the session, my client might reveal that the sinus congestion not mentioned before had disappeared. Did that mean that I had failed at the knee? Of course not! We may not necessarily know what results Reiki might bring. We never do harm sharing Reiki. We just can't control it!

As I have released my perceived "control" of the gift of Reiki, I have learned to identify and work on giving up control in other parts of my life. By striving to be the best I can be, without control, doors open and answers are revealed.

The joy in life is to be used for a purpose.
I want to be used up when I die.
—George Bernard Shaw

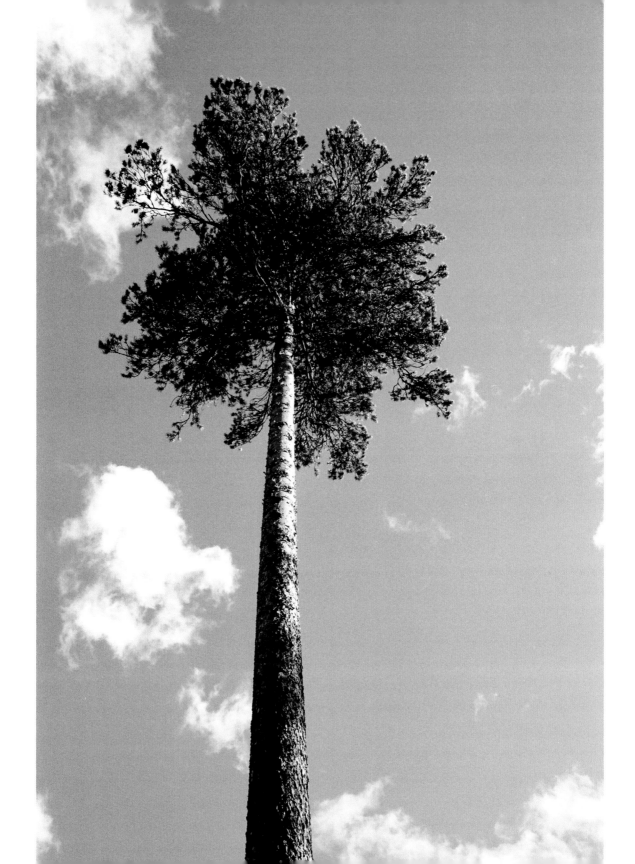

There is a difference between healing and curing. To heal is to change. To cure is to remove, make whole. Reiki heals by changing the energy that flows through the body. Reiki improves the vibrations of each organ, each tissue. Reiki may not shrink the tumor, but it will reduce the pain caused by the tumor, allowing the surrounding area to vibrate the best it can.

Reiki is promoted for the sick. Whether broken, dying, or emotionally hurting, Reiki is an excellent tool for improving the condition of life. Even though the Western medical community has been slow to discover the benefits of Reiki, as a society we are gradually demanding more, non-intrusive tools to handle our health needs. Just where acupuncture was twenty years ago, Reiki is today. With the same concept of energy movement as acupuncture, Reiki is another method of application.

When pain is a result of the "cure," it has been easier to introduce Reiki. The discomfort of chemotherapy has warranted the use of Reiki during the administering as well as afterwards, because the effects of the poison change the vibrations of the body. We can float away from the nausea and pain experienced during chemo while Reiki is gently shared.

Pregnancy and delivery can also be less stressful and less painful if Reiki is included in the care. As body parts stretch and become ready for delivery, we marvel, sometimes in fear, at what is happening to our bodies. Our fears and pains can be minimized with regular Reiki.

Heart or orthopedic rehabilitation is more successful if additional tools are offered to help ease the body back to health after surgery. Emotional adjustments as well as body limits are enhanced with a course of Reiki. Reiki may not repair a leaky heart valve, but the healing of the body and the soul can be accelerated with pre- and post-surgery sessions.

It is evident that Reiki supports recovery. But what about those who believe they are "healthy?" As I like to say, "I have never met a living thing (or person, I guess) who would not benefit from a shot of Reiki."

Life of all sorts is filled with the incomplete, the imperfect, the un-needed. We may not realize that a tree is fighting an infestation of beetles, or we may not see the hunger in the life of that rabbit, or we may think all is well within our bodies. We frantically push through life, and if we do not fall down in exhaustion, pain, or fear—well, we must be fine!

I came from the corporate world—the world where thoughts, feelings, joys, delights are squashed in honor of bottom lines, cost efficiency, competition, and survival. Some day soon we will remember that joy can improve bottom lines, cost efficiency, competition, and survival. The corporate world is but one element in our world. Let's add relationships, childcare, sports participation, bill paying, and aging parents to our world.

Making our way through life includes many assaults upon our "healthy" bodies. We struggle to keep our energy flowing smoothly, as our world expands to take on age appropriate responsibilities. If energy is blocked in parts of the body, we can pretty much count on some type of reaction ... a cold, a twinge of arthritis, or some sort of depression. No one is immune to the effects of life.

So, even the so-called healthy person can reap the benefits of Reiki. Emotional turmoil is lessened, tense muscles relax, pain diminishes, and even the unfelt mis-vibrations are addressed by sharing Reiki.

I have "healthy" friends and family. I never cease to offer Reiki. Some wonder why I mention a modality used to deal with our bodies when we are less than healthy. I maintain we all need to keep our energy flowing the best it can. We all need to let our cares go for a few minutes. We all need to soothe our souls. We all need the joy of Reiki.

Every minute should be enjoyed and savored.
—Earl Nightingale

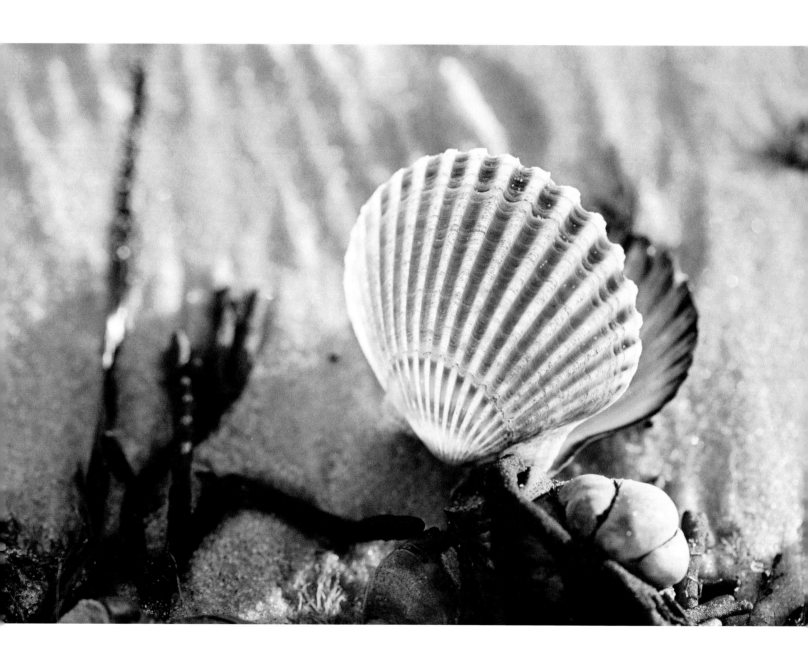

AFRAID OF FEAR

Fear is a funny word. Just saying it out loud can cause your heart to beat louder, your palms to sweat, your breathing to increase. And yet fear is a personal emotion that is controlled by our own thinking, senses, and perceptions. We can have control over our fears. We can release fear.

Fear can have multiple manifestations. It can be triggered by the nearness of danger, the expectation of pain, by the unknown, or by perceived weakness and the consequences that may occur from it.

Fear is a learned response. Not only do we learn it from our environment, but we also gather fears from our experiences, our peers, and our knowledge. Whoever said fear is eliminated with knowledge never watched the news on television. Learning how disease travels doesn't stop us from worrying about the flu season. Alerting us to the fact that there even is a flu season doesn't put our fears of illness to rest, but learning how to eat wisely, sleep appropriately, and wash vigorously reduces those fears.

There can be a fear of Reiki, whether you are the practitioner or the client. It is amazing how something so beautiful can bring up feelings that make us uncomfortable.

If our energy is to run as smoothly as possible, we may have to examine feelings that are brought to the surface or that might be blocking our well being—fear of touch, feelings of sadness, fear of speaking up, performance fears. Our beings are composed of our past, present and, some say, even our future energies. We may also have feelings we are avoiding.

As a Reiki recipient, we may fear that something will "hurt" if some rearranging is going on inside. I have had clients who were afraid they might snore or drool or otherwise lose control. Stomach growling, gas passing, body twitching—all results of relaxation and energy flow—bring up performance fears. Outbursts of laughter or gentle sobs can strike fear into a client unless they understand that healing and change illicit emotional response.

In a Reiki session, fear of the unknown is perhaps the greatest fear. This is unnecessary if the practitioner has gently and thoroughly explained the process and answered any questions. I once had a healing with a practitioner who was well versed in Native American methods of energy work. Not only did she emit some strange growls and grunts, but she also abruptly placed her hands up my pant legs. Now, here I am, an experienced energy worker, and I felt a whisper of fear. Even though I knew that energy does not harm, I wondered what was going on. If I could feel that fear, how would an inexperienced client react? Perhaps the practitioner assumed I was an old hand and didn't need an explanation of her methods. That experience confirmed my belief that clients need communication, whether they are new to you, new to Reiki, or even new to a specific problem facing them. Our job as practitioners is to teach, explain, demonstrate and communicate.

I related this to another learning experience I had had when I first began working at a bank. I was a teller/trainer and eventually lost the awe I had initially felt in handling large amounts of cash. I threw bundles of money around like bags of sugar and never thought a thing about it. One of my trainees was struck almost mute with the physical proximity to this wealth. I had forgotten to discuss the responsibility, the routine, and the respect needed to execute the job well. I had not communicated the feelings that I too had felt in my early money-handling days. Fears of making a mistake, or of forgetting the proper procedures when handling money were overwhelming my trainee. Anything new, anything unknown, anything awesome can create unhealthy fears.

On the other side of the coin (former banking lingo), a Reiki practitioner can also experience fear, mostly of performance. As newly minted practitioners, we often get into our heads by thinking too deeply about exact hand placement or the perfect amount of time at each position, all the while straining to keep our thoughts focused on the client, on the energy, or on the results. At some point, we realize that time, place, and even attempts at control are all of no consequence. As new practitioners, we may also feel that we should be able to anticipate any reactions to the Reiki energy. Every once in a while, a snort, jerk, or moan might cause us to question exactly what is happening. We just need to always remember that Reiki can do no harm.

As a new practitioner, I was also afraid I wasn't giving myself Reiki correctly. No one was watching, no one was correcting, no one would know if I made "mistakes." As hard as I tried, waters did not part, trumpets did not sound, nor did I rise above the clouds in ecstasy. My performance fears rivaled those of a sixty-year-old man involved in internet dating. After I examined my fear, and then let it go, I discovered the joy in receiving Reiki from myself. I let go of expectations, rules, and control, and acknowledged the calm relaxation provided by the gentle touch of Reiki. I healed.

The mere sense of living is joy enough.
—Emily Dickinson

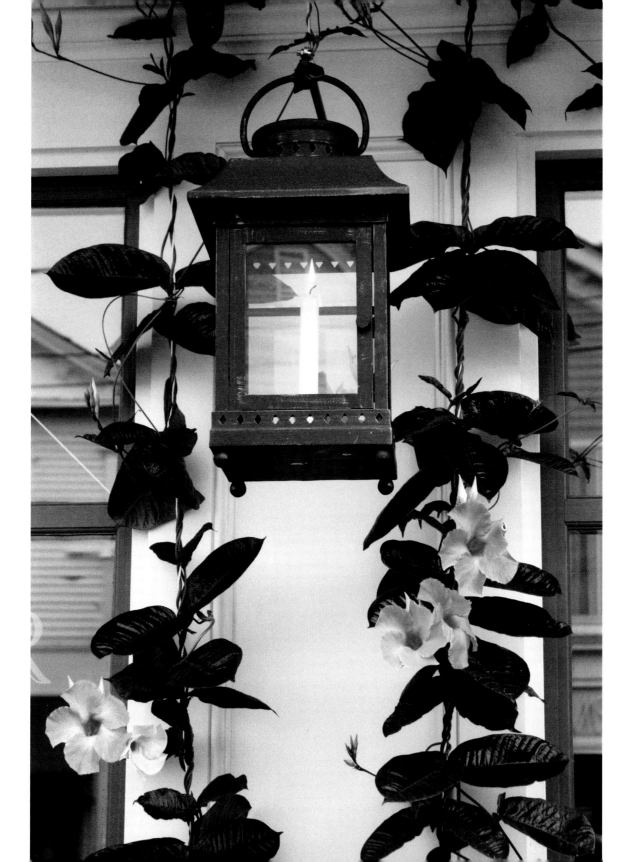

ONE LAST TOUCH

If we are honest with ourselves, most of us have had some fear connected with dying. Whether we are afraid of our own unknown future, or whether we feel helpless around the dying, each of us can claim some trepidation.

As a hospice volunteer, I have chosen to help the dying and their families. I may not have resolved my issues about death and dying, but I am on a path that will offer insight into my own personal growth.

I care. I give. I don't think a lot about dying or being with someone who is dying. I haven't gotten my story ready ... for myself or others. I have been moments away from someone's death, and I have come upon the newly departed.

I have experienced few deaths in my life that affected me intimately—and I might add that animals outnumber the humans. Because I live in the moment, death hasn't touched my reality "in the moment." Only reflection or future concerns give me pause.

As a hospice Reiki volunteer, I share the joy of offering the peace found in Reiki energy. I acknowledge the awe of giving a patient the opportunity to be the best he can be at that moment. Stress dissolves; calm prevails; nausea disappears; pain dissipates. Reiki is an excellent tool to enhance medicine and spirit alike.

As a patient nears death, issues may rise to the surface that inhibit the transitional path. Fear, bitterness, anger, and loss of control can create roadblocks at the end of one's life journey. Reiki, in its perfect form, can prepare us for the change that we call death.

Today I gave Reiki to a hospice patient as she died. I experienced her last breath; I felt her energy fade. I thought I was unprepared, and yet, it was the most natural experience I could imagine.

When I arrived, the house was full of commotion. Daughters, sons-in-law, great-grandkids, phones, televisions, computers ... no calm was blanketing this home. I entered as a stranger (I was "subbing" for another volunteer) and had been asked to give Reiki to a daughter who was emotionally adrift and in need of a calming touch. I was not planning to see Nora, the hospice patient and mother of the daughter I was scheduled to see.

When I arrived, the daughter was not ready for me and was showering after a rough morning with Nora (who had been out of bed and was alert, I might add). A son-in-law directed me to Nora's room instead, to "work on her." Another daughter was in the room, watching television. Nora was awake and I introduced myself, saying I was here as her Reiki practitioner and began Reiki. I marveled out loud at the beauty of her room and at the wonderful family who surrounded her. At this point the family left the room and turned off the TV, even though I had urged them to do whatever they wished.

Nora was a bit restless, moaning at exhale, fidgeting under the blankets. I closed my eyes to center myself and began taking stock of my senses. I noticed a movement from the patient, and as I opened my eyes, she was struggling to reach a glass of water. I ended the Reiki and helped her drink a few sips. As I started again, I sensed her body relax, and as I glanced at my watch, I felt that a half hour session would be beneficial.

Without warning, as the half hour mark arrived, the patient, who was propped up in bed, rose up a bit, and with her eyes open, took a few deep breaths, lay back down and died.

There had been no struggle, no fear, no gasping sounds. As she had risen up, I had continued Reiki, and had repeated, "It's all right, it's all right," until her head reclined back on the pillow. Once she fell back, I studied her chest for breaths (I saw a slight movement) and decided that perhaps I should get the family in the room.

I stepped out of the room and motioned to the daughter who had asked for Reiki, remembering that we had not yet met. She came into my arms in the hallway and I whispered without forethought, "Your mother's breathing pattern has changed and you might want to come into the room." She went to the door and immediately noted that Nora's color had changed. She turned back to me and clutched me with emotion. She asked me to get her sister. The three of us sat in the Nora's room as I continued to give Reiki to her. When the medically experienced daughter checked her mother, she was confident that she had died. I still wasn't sure, and didn't want to make any assumptions. My response was. "Shall I step out of the room?" I suggested a call to hospice.

The daughters wanted me to stay in the house. I became the "babysitter" to the grandkids as they watched *Free Willie* and played *Barbie Computer*. I continued to Reiki the house. In doing so, I listened to the chatter of cell phones and to somber phone calls, and I felt a calm descend. Although muffled sobs intermittently rose above the hum of activity, the racing around and almost-hysteria disappeared. It was as if a gentle hand were at everyone's elbow, guiding each family member in his grief and activities.

After the family's hospice nurse arrived and made the necessary exam and contacts, we quietly sat in the kitchen. There was a sense of peace. I stayed with the family until I felt that it was time to leave.

I left the house to encounter a huddle of family members quietly talking in the sea of cars. My car was blocked in, but the home-owning son-in-law urged me to drive across the yard, if necessary. As I maneuvered my small convertible out of the drive, I felt the urge to lower the top. I was feeling that something big needed to be released. Once away from the house, I drove down the country road, top down, music blaring, releasing the spirit of connection. I was at peace.

The ride back to town gave me time to review the wondrous events of the past hours. While I was an unknown to the family, they had embraced my visit and its outcome with love and gratitude. Each phone call had included, "it's over … she died peacefully … she is no longer in pain … the Reiki Lady was here."

One last touch.

Since you get more joy out of giving joy to others, you should put a good deal of thought into the happiness that you are able to give.

—Eleanor Roosevelt

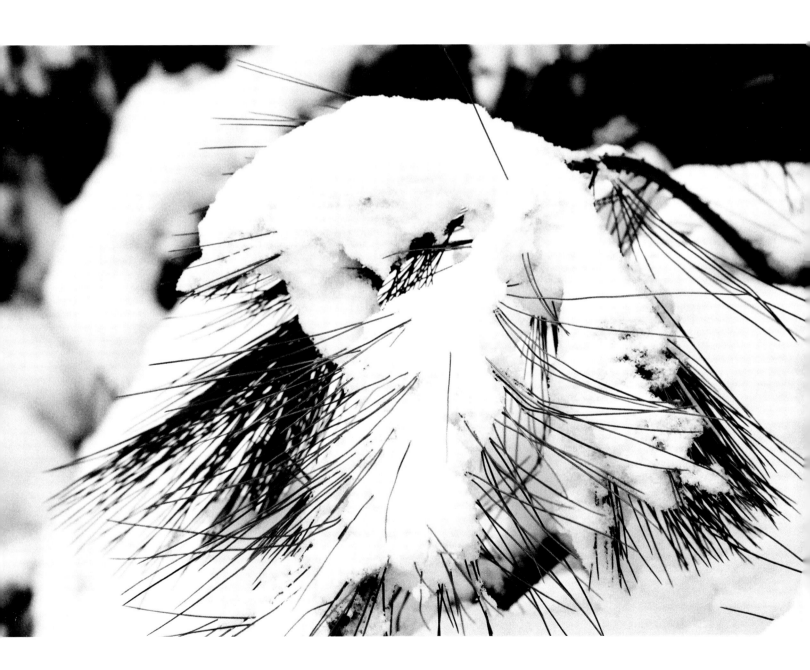

THE SANTA EFFECT

Santa Claus was explained to me at Christmas one year. I was in the second grade, some say a bit young to grasp the difference between a red-suited jolly man and the spirit of the season.

My parents quietly asked me into the kitchen on Christmas evening while my younger sisters and older brother continued reveling around our heavily decorated tree. I don't remember what exactly was said. I am sure all the proper words were spoken to ensure my continued faith in the unseen joy of the holiday. My parents wanted me to hear the story from them before my friends shared any news. They also entreated me to protect the innocence of my sisters who were significantly younger.

I was wrapped up in the fact that my parents, as Santa, had given me my first watch, a Timex. It glowed in the dark — I suppose for all the times that I would leave it on at night to track the passage of time. I was amazed that my parents, who were traditionally fiscally sound, would throw caution to the wind and share such bounty with their child. That watch began my shift into "grown-up thinking." I felt honored that I was old enough to accept this responsibility. This first watch met the full bathtub one too many times, often

sailed to the ground accidentally, and was scratched and dented at the end. I kept that watch for years. A sign of growing up.

Although I questioned the mechanics of the news about Santa, I trusted my parent's knowledge. I was amazed that Santa's gifts, when wrapped, bore paper unlike anything else under the tree; our stockings contained appropriate gifts wrapped in yet another type of wrapping; and any gifts addressed to any one of us had tags written in a mysterious handwriting. I later discovered this to be my mother's use of her left hand as an attempt to disguise the author. (I was sharp enough, however, to also ask about the origins of the Easter Bunny and the Tooth Fairy at this same heart-to-heart.)

The joy and wonder of the holidays were not diminished for me. The unveiling of the gift procurers did nothing to dampen my youthful enthusiasm for the magic of gift receiving. I still had the anticipation of marching down the stairs Christmas morning, youngest first, to a room full of magic.

I continue to enjoy receiving gifts. As I have matured, I have learned to look for gifts in all of life — a beautiful sunrise, a gurgling baby's smile, an unexpected card in the mail (so much more surprising than an appropriate e-card). The feeling can best be described as a tingle of connection with what is given, plus the surprise, joy, and acknowledgement of the gift—certainly this must be Santa Claus at his best!

Reiki does that for me. At first, I sought results as gifts to my abilities. If a client smiled, felt a reduction in pain, or dozed after a night of insomnia, I was pleased I could give such a gift. Some clients saw visions, had emotional breakthroughs, or marveled at the sense of calm that washed over them.

At the same time, I felt that each recipient of Reiki was a gift to me. I felt such respect and honor as I was allowed to step into the private energy of each client. There were days when tears came to my eyes as a client breathed thanks. I tried to explain to them that they too gave me a gift because I was receiving the same energy they were. I became the best I could be as I shared Universal Life Force Energy, that big, amazing, all encompassing power of healing, with them.

At this stage of my life, I realize that Santa had as much fun giving as I did receiving. He spent a lot of time pouring over lists, replaying conversations, staying vigilant in a child's sharing of dreams. He made secret and mysterious trips, found various hiding places, and chuckled in anticipation of the day. Could he actually have had more fun than I? Maybe so—he had more time to feel the tingle.

Today I try to tingle with the Santa Effect daily. It takes an awareness of your surroundings, an opening of your heart, and an acknowledgement of the gifts around you. I send energy to those in need, whether friend or stranger. I touch what is available in Nature. I give the gift of caring to others and receive the tingle.

Surely joy is the condition of life.
—Henry David Thoreau

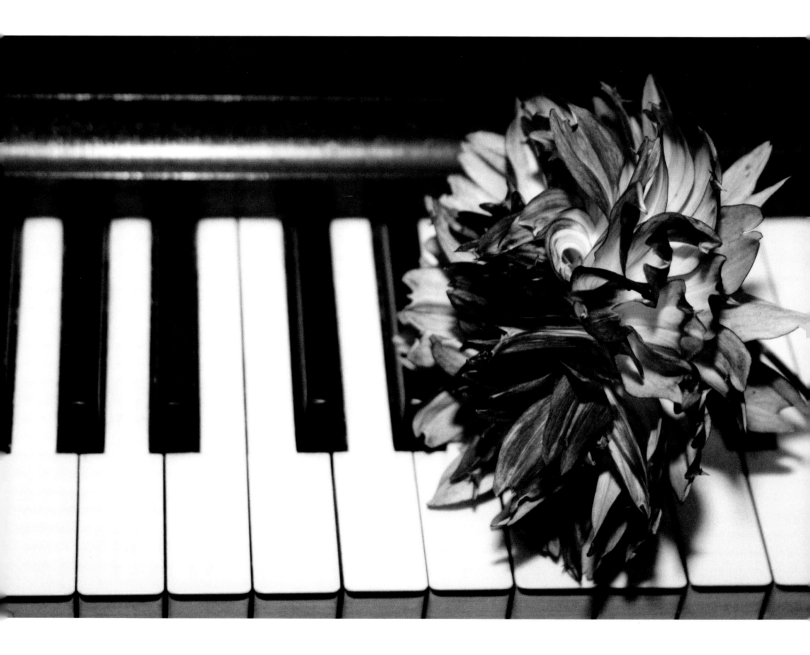

I HEAR MUSIC

It fascinates me that everything is connected. It took me many years to become aware of the fabric of life. It doesn't take a special religion, a scientific study, or years of experience to come to this conclusion. It takes only moments of reflection to determine that we all are connected by air, water, energy, and spirit.

In our special relationship to the dimension or the plane in which we live, we "see," "hear," and "taste" the vibrations that make up our lives. We sleep on the best beds we can create, we eat food that we find attractive to our lifestyles, we hear music in nature, from our Ipods, and occasionally in concert. The vibrations of life resonate with the vibrations of our bodies.

Our individuality determines our needs. I live quite simply. From age, life situation, and my scale of beauty, I have few possessions. I have found peace in my choice of home, city, and part of the country in which I live. My vibrations hum the best in the Heartland, it seems, but my soul remains by the water. I am content with that duality.

I have always required music in my life. Music is my escape, my meditation, my joy. My home is cleaner with a pulsing bass throbbing to the beat of my scrubbing (although the scrubbing doesn't happen nearly as often as the pulsing bass). Sundays are more spiritual with classical music drifting to my ear. I cannot imagine reading the Sunday New York Times without the formality of a symphony in the background. My car trips are shorter and easier with Motown streaming out of my speakers. I live through music.

I relished the concept of accompanying Reiki sessions with soft New Age music, weaving a connection of energy to the client and to the practitioner. I felt it was necessary to set a mood for a Reiki experience, and I believed the music was for the client. I soon discovered that the music was for me. The best Reiki experience does not need music, but I continue to find the most joy when music is involved with the energy.

Often, I bring music to homebound clients. I try to create an oasis of relaxation. The music masks phones ringing, dishes slapping against each other, heavy footsteps carrying on the daily routine. I may rotate musical selections until I discover the client's preference in the connection of music with relax-ation. My clients have varying tastes—what soothes one may jar another's sensibilities. I have had clients choose golden oldies, country, or even jazz as a musical relaxation tool, a demonstration of how one chooses particular vibrations that resonate within the individual.

Here is my conclusion. It brings science, spirit, and Stinnett philosophies together. Once I discover a client's particular choice of relaxation music, I give him a copy of it. That music vibrates specifically for him ... for him to be the best he can be while relaxing. If I were to share Reiki while that music is playing, his body would learn to identify the feelings experienced with Reiki with that music. Cellular memories could be triggered by the vibrations he received from those particular songs. The sense of peace, the reduction of pain, the lessening of fears could actually occur from hearing that music.

Does Reiki begin without the practitioner when the music plays? No, but the body remembers the calm it experienced when Reiki was shared. The body has the opportunity to become the best it can be in that moment. The connection between the vibrations of the music and that person's individual vibrations is made.

Since music is in nature, we all have access to vibrations that allow us to relax, to remember, to meditate. The whisper of the breeze stroking the trees, the gentle beat of rain on the roof, or the movement of the lake.... What delightful vibrations.

Music can heal. Music can connect. Music can be everywhere.

Our goal should be to achieve joy.
—Ana Castillo

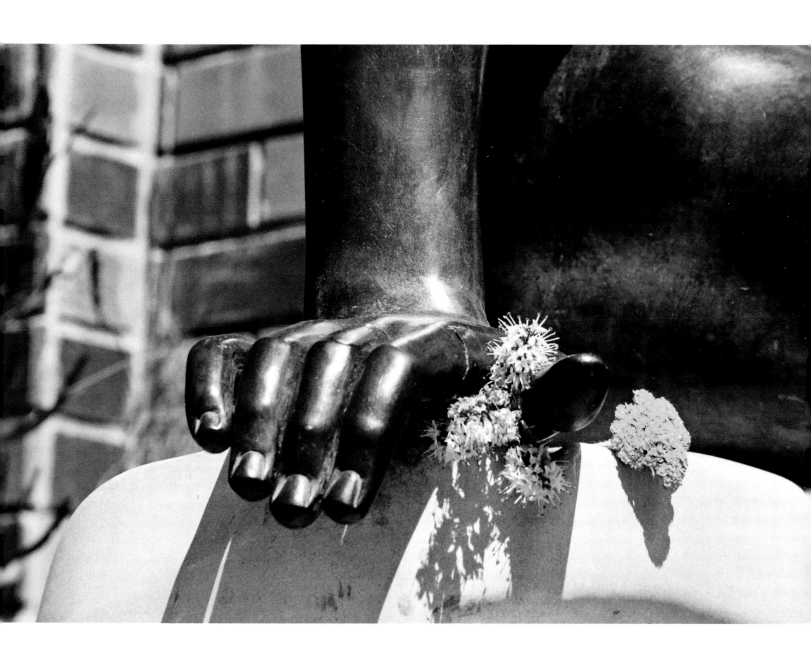

Words are an important means of communication. We share our innermost thoughts and feelings through the spoken or written word. It is interesting to note, however, that there can be different ways of expressing the same meaning, and there can be different ways of interpreting the same words. Our day-to-day world is filled with crossover meanings. A sigh—not exactly a word—can express contentment or frustration.

At times we do not use the correct word to express an exact feeling, and sometimes our choice of a word sends an entirely different message to the listener. Some hear the word as it is meant while others hear something entirely different.

And so it is with Reiki. Reiki falls under an umbrella that struggles to identify what it covers. Why, even the umbrella is referred to by using different terms. No wonder everyone is confused. In its early Western existence, Reiki was an Alternative. Alternative could mean "instead of," and those who followed its practice never felt that Reiki could replace all the benefits of medicine rooted in chemistry and physics. By identifying Reiki as a Complimentary Modality, some believed it to be a "no cost for service." One of the longest standing monikers is Complimentary/Alternative Medicine or CAM.

CAM employed that mysterious term "medicine." Professionals kept adding items under the CAM umbrella—nutrition, exercise, and aromatherapy.... The lists lengthened and the number of questions increased. How could eating in a certain way be classified as medicine?

The term Alternative has slipped away in popularity to be replaced with Integrative—an intention that "includes" rather than "excludes." That concept supports the thought that one can use tools from many modalities to manage the mind, body, and spirit. And by dividing one's being into these three areas, another completely diverse way of treating our health is created.

Therapy ... medicine ... technique.... What is your choice? It really doesn't matter.

Within the practice of Reiki there are different terms and paths. Some students are attuned to the energy, while some are initiated. Both terms explain the opening of energy paths. Every student experiences a shift that allows him to access Universal Life Force Energy. And what about that term? Some equate Universal Life Force Energy with Spirit or God. I believe that to compare religion and Reiki is like comparing cars to kittens. Both move, both can bring joy, but each is a different tool used to find joy.

Some practitioners are trained to keep their hands above the body. Some feel touch is an integral part of the process. Some start their session at the head, some at the feet. Some pray out loud. Some seek guidance from guides or spirits. Some intuitively see blockages; some are drawn to specific areas of the body.

Sacred symbols are another point of expression. Some believe they are secret. Some believe anyone can see them, but unless attuned or initiated, we cannot be effective with them. And while we are on the subject, when comparing symbols with other practitioners, one often finds different interpretations. Does that make them wrong? Of course not. Using the symbols you were attuned to is like saying "goin" in Alabama.... That is what you were taught, that is what you hear, and everyone understands you just fine!

My point is this: Don't get mired in the details. Don't let your head get in the way of your heart. The intention of Reiki is to relax and relieve, to calm and to heal. How we employ the therapy/technique/modality is an individual choice. We all come to Reiki with different talents, backgrounds, and abilities. We need to remember that the energy is the same.

Learning to live in the present moment
is part of the path of joy.
—Sarah Ban Breathnach

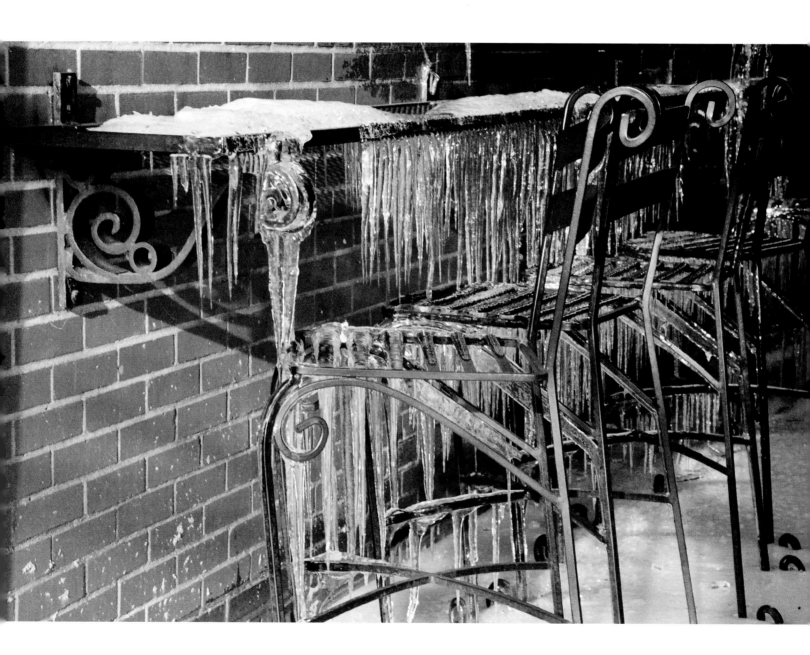

LISTENING

Many people love to talk and are good at it. Many people try to listen, but fail to grasp the concept. We are a society attached at the hip to all sorts of communication technologies, and yet, we don't always hear what is being communicated.

We start life with a strong ability to listen. We are drawn to musical notes, some say, in utero. We mimic the language we hear until we can form the appropriate words. We absorb education, of many sorts, as if we were listening sponges.

At some point, our lives may become too complicated to listen. Then all the communication technologies take over. We text, IM, cell phone, and iPod ourselves to communication nirvana, but we often lose our listening skills along the way.

At times we are encouraged to listen. Love can tap into our listening skills. Fear can create a greater need to listen, just as it might conceal what we need to hear. My favorite reason for beginning to listen again is because of life experience, or, if you are so inclined, you might call that "age." As we mature, we acknowledge that we do not have all the answers and

that others might be carrying around items of importance. And sometimes we even slow down enough to hear the beauty of running water, chirping birds, and the rustling of leaves in the trees.

As we age, we realize that we are overflowing with experiences, some to share and some to secretly smile over. We also realize that we have the time and intelligence to bring out and dust off our listening skills. Some will say they have always listened and benefited. I, however, am in the group who needed to be reminded of how to listen and what listening can do for personal growth.

While I was in college, I contracted meningitis. With the possibility of death hanging over me, I eventually walked away with only a hearing loss in my left ear. What was I not hearing? Later in life, I suffered from Menieres Disease in the same left ear ... again, not listening? I review those times in my life to determine what I was not paying attention to. Pretty basic, very telling.

For much of my adult life, I suffered from Raynaud's Phenomenon. Some of my fingertips and toes would turn white in the cold. I thought it was from a youth of ice-skating too long at the lake on those lazy winter days. It lessened as I "listened" to my body and incorporated Reiki into my daily life. I felt more heart-fully. I acknowledged that connection brought warmth.

When I lose an important document, when I can't remember what I promised a friend, when I want to open myself to the alternatives of a situation, I use Reiki. I use Reiki to lessen the impact of frustration, anger, or fear. Reiki puts me into an open state that allows me to open my mind and my heart.

Reiki helps slow down the frenetic beat of our lives. Reiki minimizes the static surrounding our consciousness. Reiki sharpens hearing, sight, and taste. In effect, it allows us to be as aware of our surroundings as when we were babies.

More importantly, Reiki allows individuals to talk, feel, communicate, and experience. As practitioners, we need to listen to what we hear, see, and feel, not only within ourselves during energy sharing, but we also need to listen to those we work with.

The client who is sick or actively dying has much to say. Reiki often opens these lines of communication better than any phone or computer. As our bodies become the best they can be, we relax and take note of all the experiences we have had or are having. Some memories are examined and shared, while others are allowed to blow away. Some insights can be appreciated and accepted. Certain sounds vibrate in tune to our bodies.

At times, the practitioner's hands become the listening tool as energy is shared. We are able to determine blocks or unrest. We might be sensitive to pain or disease. We are there to offer Reiki energy to relax and smooth the rough edges of life. We listen to the body.

As the practitioner listens, he has the opportunity to learn, appreciate, and comfort the individual. The practitioner's experiences enrich his own life and practice. A Reiki practitioner is often privy to the most personal thoughts. We need to understand what is asked of us in each setting. Listening is the greatest gift to give to another. We do not need to be in a rush to give our opinions or tell our own stories. We do not need to give our impressions of the client's status. We are there to be the sounding board. We are there to touch. We are there to listen.

Silence is the perfectest herald of joy.
　　　　　　　　　　　　—William Shakespeare

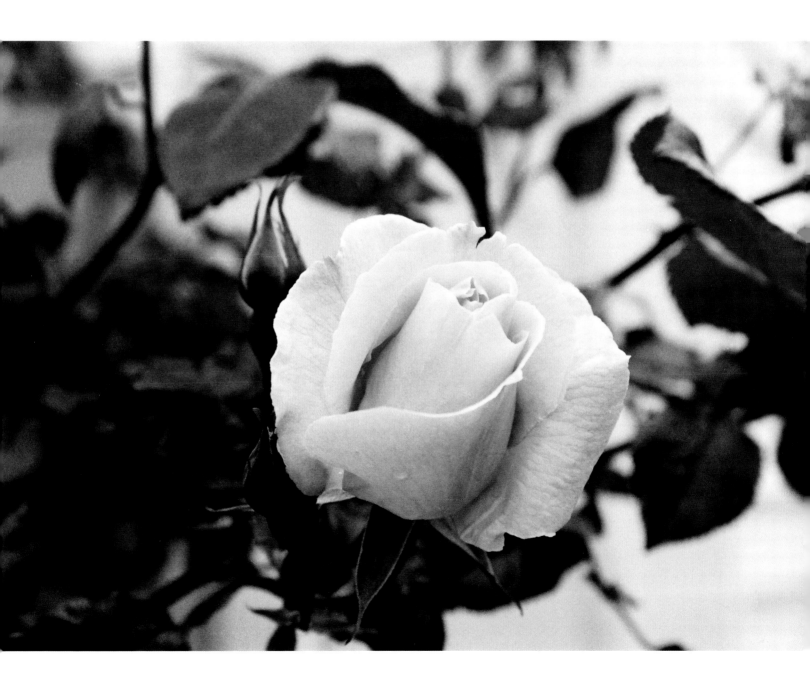

Nursing homes exist to provide the care that families once offered to the sick or dying family member. While we look with pride at the advanced and around-the-clock services available to our loved ones, we know that our lives are made easier if the necessary custodial support comes in the form of a nursing home.

I have been in a number of nursing homes. Some give me the urge to finish my business and leave. Others bring a sense of peace as I walk through the doors. In each facility that I have visited, there seems to be at least one caregiver who restores my faith in the off-site care of our loved ones.

Often I pass room after room with a heavy heart. So many residents sit alone with no visitor. Each day is an endless sea of boredom. No wonder so many fade away from this life soon after being admitted into this future of nothingness. I wish we could rectify the situation.

Small town nursing facilities seem to bring a spirit of home into the walls of the institution. You can see a more laid back, home-like environment as the aids banter and administer to the needs of their charges.

Perhaps a festival from the past weekend or a boyfriend's latest antics may be clucked over as the news of the day.

Many times I see family members of all ages attending to the personal needs of residents. This close attention may come from a strong sense of family, or from living in close proximity the nursing home. Small town living often affords one the time to be an "angel of care."

I enjoy visiting my clients in nursing homes. Smaller community homes never fail to bring me to heart-center. Usually my clients are patients of hospice and are slipping away gradually. Often the client shows few signs of an eminent end to his life, so often my nursing home clients can remain in my life for months.

Mary was one such lady who lay sweetly and quietly in bed for weeks. She never woke during my sessions, and rather often caused me to strain to see any rise in her chest from breathing. Her room was full of hand-made bedding (quilts, afghans, pillowcases), and every surface supported a family picture. I often wandered the room, either before or after my visit, absorbing the energy that these smiling, active people brought into the room, and I caressed the handmade covers draping the couch and chairs.

Mary was blessed to have a daughter living nearby, who would often be with us as I gave Reiki to her mother. The family believed that Mary was much calmer because of the energy offered through our sessions. The daughter and I formed a comfortable relationship, and I eagerly looked forward to hearing stories about her mother's past, or updates on any recent waking moments. Her visits added warmth to the room, and I watched Mary as she subtly responded to our voices and conversation.

On this particular day, Mary and I were alone. Although I usually stay at the feet of sleeping patients, that day I felt drawn to sit at her shoulders, placing her hand in mine. If I saw any movement, I would quietly remind her who I was and what I was doing. We sat in peace for a number of minutes. Again I felt a connection as Reiki caressed her fragile body. Suddenly she opened her eyes, displaying a startling clarity. A sense of wonderment came to her, and she murmured, "You are so beautiful."

Although I like to think I can still turn a head or two, I immediately realized that my client was not seeing me, but rather seeing the beauty of the moment, the sharing of the joy and calm she found in Reiki. Rather than rambling on about the state of my hair or my lack of makeup, I took the moment for what it was and gently squeezed her hand, whispering, "Thank you." She smiled a soft smile and returned to her dreams. I was in a dream of my own.

Joy is not in things, it is in us.
—Richard Wagner

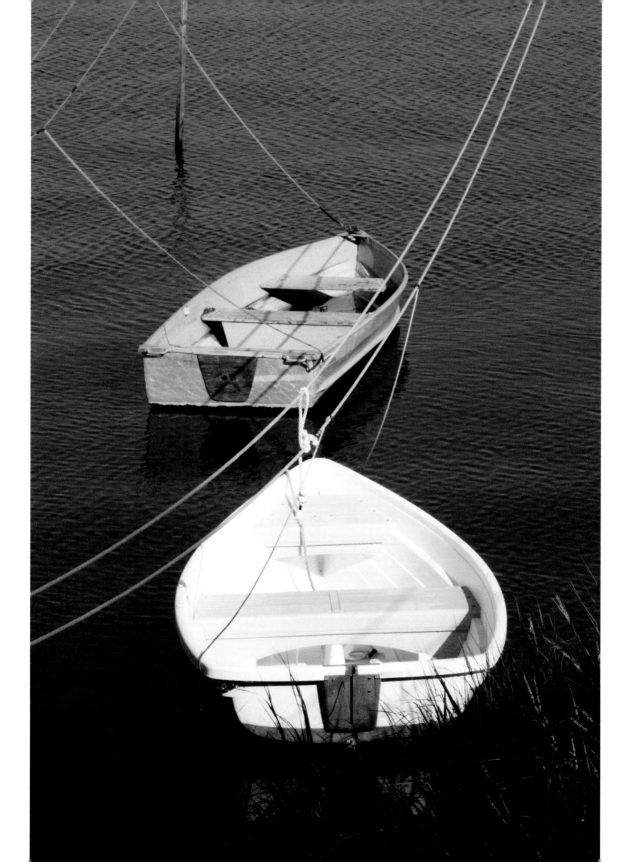

As you walk through life, you may have noticed that, at times, you walk with purpose, and at other times, wandering can best explain your forward motion. Don't let anyone tell you anything different. We all are moving forward, if only in age.

As we progress, in different ways and at different speeds, from time to time we employ tools that help us along the path. Education and knowledge, food and drink … these are among our most basic needs. What about that which makes us happy, safe, or strong? We all use different methods or techniques to help keep us the best we can be.

I have friends who get "high" on a treadmill. Some of the most beautiful smiles can be found after a religious service. We feel the energy generated after a rock concert. We observe the glow on a professor's face after a rousing lecture. Most of us can identify what it is that improves our existence. It may be diet, prayer, music, books, or exercise. It may be all of these or a unique combination that suits the soul. It may be approved or unapproved substances. It may be new experiences or repetition.

I believe that intention is the key to being the best we can be. If we visualize a healthy heart, that treadmill will serve its purpose. If we relax to Yo-Yo Ma, a cello sighting could lower our heart rate. Our intention to be the best we can be may take many forms. We must listen to our hearts to discover our path.

Joy has two components for me. When I experience joy, not only do I feel it, but those around me do as well. I experience joy, by sharing, giving, helping, and being of service. I know that when I feel my best, I feel joy.

I believe in energy and I believe we are connected through energy. I believe Reiki energy brings joy to the practitioner and to the recipient. I believe we are the best we can be when sharing Reiki. I believe that through love, prayer, intention, thought, and meditation, everything is connected. What goes around comes around. You get what you give. Do unto others as you would have them do unto you…. Get the drift?

For me, there are many ways to discover joy. I have found my way. May you find yours. I hope your joy includes receiving as well as giving, and that your joy provides peace, calm, happiness, understanding, abundance … love.

Please take a moment to identify your joy and know that in being the best you can be, you will share that joy. Incorporate joy daily. Be thankful and smile. You are blessed.

The aim of life is to live and to live means to be aware, joyously drunkenly, serenely, divinely aware.
—Henry Miller

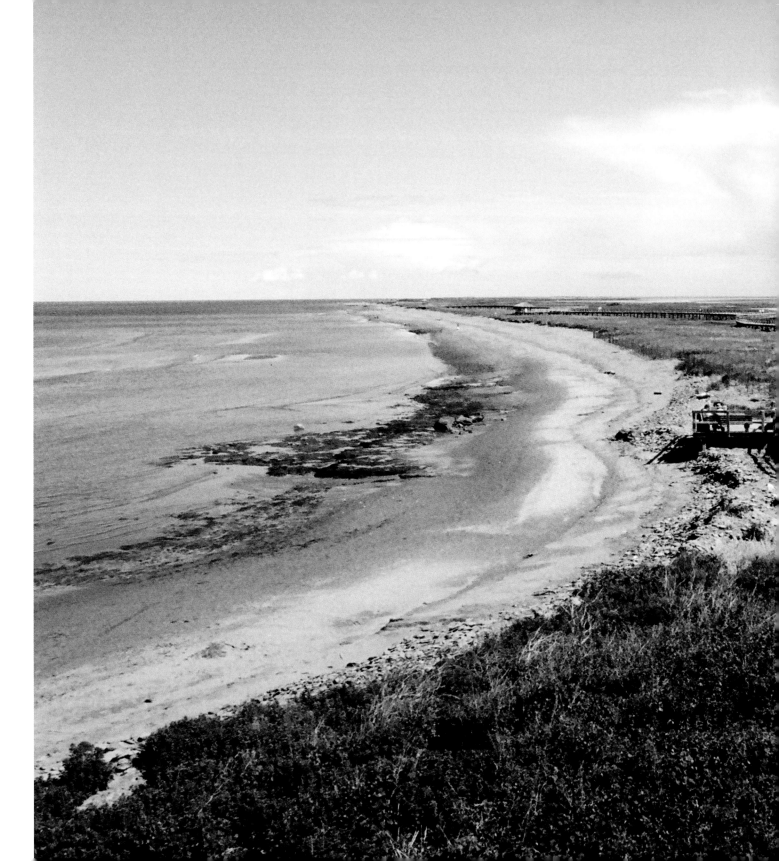

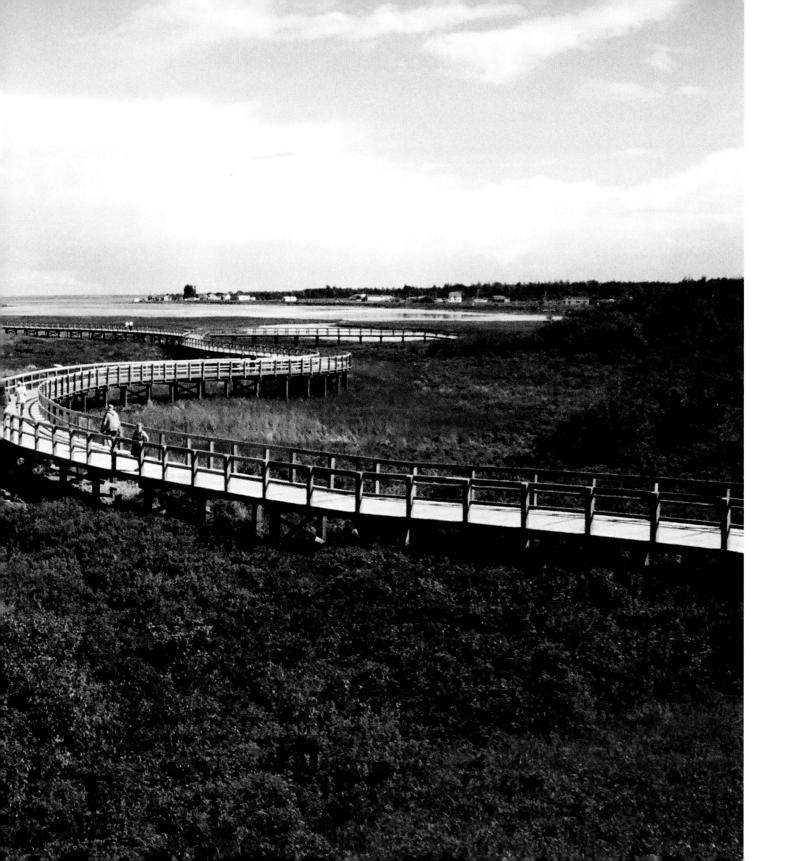

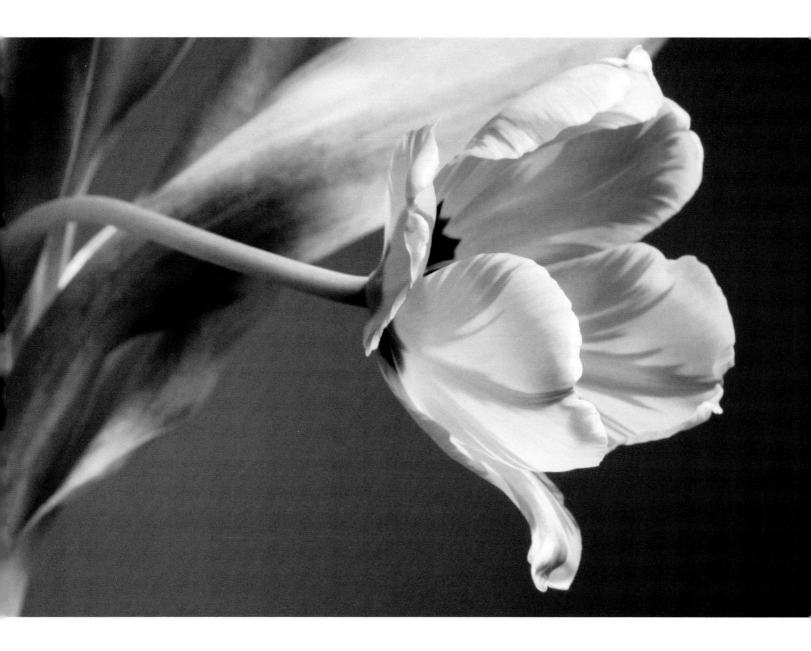

PHOTOGRAPHS

ACKNOWLEDGMENTS

I feel as if I am at the Academy Awards. I am standing in front of hundreds (well, millions, if you count the television watchers). I am unfolding my scrap of paper clutched in my fist. I am fearful of forgetting some-one important. I am stunned to be here. I am choked up with emotion. I begin.

I want to thank my family, those with me today and those who have departed, whose support is the foundation of all that I am.

I thank my best friends and my husbands, at times one and the same, but varied over the years.

I offer tribute to my teachers and mentors, whether academic, career, experience, or spiritual, who influenced my participation in life.

I appreciate the willingness of various hospital, hospice, and nursing facilities in Illinois and Connecticut to share in providing opportunities for my growth.

I thank my clients and patients who swell the experience factor, with some trickling into the friend category.

And that just gets me to this book. I thank Carin Roaldset, photographer extraordinaire and my trusted and delightful editors and publishers, Nancy Stem and Kay Fowler. Where would I be without the beauty, guidance, and experience shared during this process?

My inclusion frenzy grows. Perhaps now is the moment to explain my theory of personal energy. Each of us carries energy from every person who has impacted our life, whether family, lover, friend, or stranger. Situations and events can add energy that molds our beliefs and morals.

Therefore, I take this moment to thank every person who has touched my soul and every situation that has provided a lesson for me in order that I might share my stories with you.

Thank you.

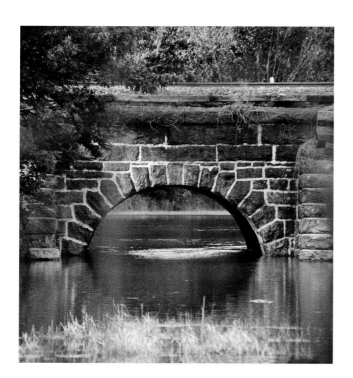

THE BRANFORD FOUNDATION

Funds for the printing and distribution of this book are provided by The Branford Foundation. This charitable organization provides a variety of Integrative Therapy programs, materials, and services to the community. The health of each participant is affected by the expertise of those who volunteer and participate in the foundation's efforts. To learn more about the impact and potential of The Branford Foundation and to discover how you can help, please refer to www.thebranfordfoundation.org.